BASIC INSTINCTS

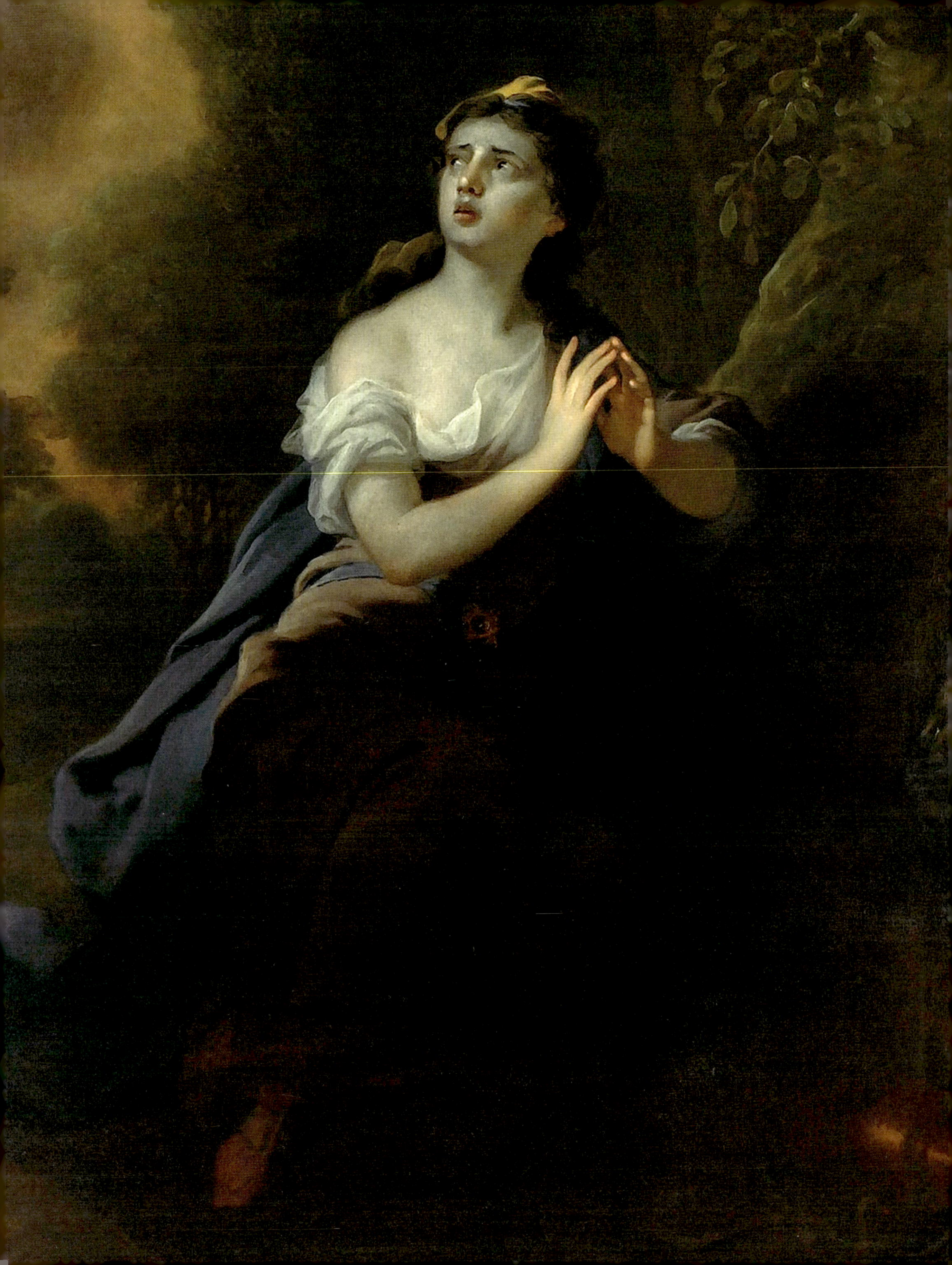

BASIC INSTINCTS

Love, Passion and Violence in the Art of Joseph Highmore

JACQUELINE RIDING

PAUL HOLBERTON PUBLISHING

First published to accompany the exhibition *Basic Instincts* at the Foundling Museum, London, 29 September 2017 – 7 January 2018

ISBN 978 1 911300 28 1

British Library Catalogue in Publishing Data

A CIP record of this publication is available from the British Library

Produced by Paul Holberton Publishing
89 Borough High St, London SE1 1NL
WWW.PAULHOLBERTON.COM

Designed by Laura Parker

Printed by Ganboa Centro Gráfico, Spain

FRONT COVER Joseph Highmore, *The Angel of Mercy*, c.1746 (detail of fig. 94)
BACK COVER Joseph Highmore, *Susanna Highmore*, c.1740–45 (detail of fig. 9)

LOWELL
LIBSON LTD
BRITISH ART

CONTENTS

FOREWORD

In December 1816 James Caulfield wrote to an unnamed individual regarding a painting in his possession which he described as 'Hogarth's first design on the subject of the Foundling Hospital'. The purpose of the letter was to remind the recipient of Caulfield's offer to bring the work 'to the notice of the Governors of the Institution'. Caulfield goes on to say that Hogarth's canvas 'represents an imprudent mother about to strangle her offspring but is prevented from the crime by the interposition of an Angel, who points to the Asylum of the Foundling, as a sanctuary, – while the nurse is retiring evidently affected by the scene'. Caulfield then observes that Hogarth 'abandoned Allegory for Scripture' and instead 'painted Moses as the First Foundling on record', a reference to the artist's gift to the hospital, *Moses brought before Pharaoh's Daughter*, of 1746. Caulfield concludes, 'the price I value it at is Eighty Guineas, which I trust will be considered a moderate charge both in respect to the merit of the Painting and the rarity of this great Artists works'.[1]

Caulfield's offer was clearly rejected by the hospital's governors, as a century and a half later the painting emerged at Sotheby's London saleroom. Still attributed to Hogarth, the murderous actions of the 'imprudent mother' are now glossed over with the description 'An Angel succouring a foundling child .... Said to be a sketch for the altarpiece of the Foundling Hospital'.[2] Six years on, at Christie's 'Important English Pictures' sale, the painting was still considered to be a design by Hogarth for the Foundling Hospital altarpiece, but had now acquired a title, *The Angel of Mercy* (front cover, fig. 94).[3]

This painting was bought at the sale by Colnaghi and soon after acquired by Paul Mellon. It remains, as part of Paul Mellon's gift, at the Yale Center for British Art. No doubt the attribution to William Hogarth, the most famous and highly valued British artist working in the early Georgian period, was a crucial factor in its purchase. The attribution was accepted by the Hogarth scholar Ronald Paulson, who included it in his magisterial *Hogarth, His Life, His Art and Times* (1971).[4]

However, the suggestion put forward by Dr Brian Allen (then Director of the Paul Mellon Centre in London) that, rather than by Hogarth, the painting was by Joseph Highmore (1692–1780), Hogarth's exact contemporary and an artist, likewise associated with London's Foundling Hospital, is now universally accepted and this reattribution, based predominantly on style, has been supported by additional research.[5] The story of *The Angel of Mercy*'s journey from Highmore to Hogarth to Highmore is a salutary reminder of the vagaries of attribution. From the early nineteenth century, the desire for the painting to be by Hogarth seems to have overridden key evidence suggesting the contrary, not least the painting itself, although it is understandable that the prime candidate for such a disturbing scene would be the creator of 'A Harlot's Progress' and 'Marriage A-la Mode' rather than a little-known portrait painter. Highmore's celebrated group portrait *Mr Oldham and his Guests* (Tate) has a similar history, and its attribution to Hogarth, like *The Angel of Mercy*, had occurred within decades of Highmore's death. The reattribution of the latter to a 'lesser' – that is less commercially attractive – artist, may explain why such an extraordinary painting has received so little attention until now.

As this publication will reveal, *The Angel of Mercy* (cover and fig. 94) deserves our attention. Over the following chapters, the painting will be placed within both the broader context of Highmore's life and art and, specifically, given the painting's particular subject-matter, his approach to family and mother-and-child portraiture, including examples of the artist's own wife and children; his close association with Samuel Richardson (1689–1761) and the author's tormented heroines Pamela (published 1740–41) and Clarissa (1748); and finally Highmore's connection, personally and professionally, with Britain's first children's charity, the Foundling Hospital (founded 1739). What emerges are highly contentious and emotive issues, which challenged contemporary society and directly led to *The Angel of Mercy*'s creation, such as the status and care of women and children, master/servant relations, motherhood, reputation, abuse, abandonment, infant death and new-born child murder. Inseparable from these themes are the gamut of basic human instincts, or impulses, from love – whether romantic, familial, parental or fraternal – passion, compassion and humanity, to egotism, cruelty, fear and violence.

The Angel of Mercy's presence in the exhibition signifies the first time, since its creation, that Highmore's painting has been displayed to the general public in the United Kingdom. Crucially it signals the arrival, at last, of *The Angel of Mercy* at the Foundling Hospital's site – its place of inspiration and origin – exactly two centuries after James Caulfield first proposed it.

This book has been many years in the making. It is twenty-five years since I started cataloguing Susanna Duncombe née Highmore's sketches at Tate and twenty-three years since I submitted my MA dissertation on her.[6] The daughter led me to the father.

Enormous thanks to Lowell Libson for his generous sponsorship and to the Marc Fitch Fund; to the Paul Mellon Centre, and the following institutions who either greatly reduced or completely waived their image fees: The Art Gallery of South Australia; The Fitzwilliam Museum, Cambridge; The Garrick Club, London; McMaster University Library, Ontario; The Metropolitan Museum of Art, New York; National Gallery of Victoria, Melbourne; National Portrait Gallery, London; The National Trust for England; St Bartholomew's Hospital Archive; Waddesdon Manor; Wolverhampton Art Gallery, and the Yale Centre for British Art.

Particular thanks to William Vaughan, my MA dissertation supervisor at Birkbeck College, University of London; Mark Hallett, my PhD supervisor at the University of York; Elizabeth Einberg, who introduced me to Joseph Highmore and his family; and Brian Allen, who in 1997 gave me a black-and-white photograph of *The Angel of Mercy* saying, 'This will interest you'. Their support and encouragement over many years has been greatly appreciated.

I have had the very great pleasure of corresponding with Highmore's descendants in Canada and Australia, Joan Highmore Blackhall and Amanda Jane Briedahl. My gratitude to Lord Malmesbury for giving permission to quote from his family archive and allowing me to view his very fine Highmore collection, and to the private owner of Highmore's *The Artist and his Family*; also to the following colleagues, friends and family: Tabitha Barber, Clare Barlow, Tim Batchelor, Caroline Campbell, Juliet Carey, Jane Darcy, Janet Dickinson, Helen Dorey, Sarah Fraser, John Goodall, Robin Hamlyn (who sadly died last year and is greatly missed), Matthew Hargraves, Rhian Harris, Malcolm Hay, Karen Hearn, Carmen Holdsworth-Delgado, Laura Houliston, Eleanor Hughes, Richard Humphries, Anne Lyles, Richard Johns, Johanna Marschner, Leela Meinertas, Jane Munro, Amy Myers, Steven Parissien, Caroline Pegum, Martin Postle, Eileen Read, Kate Retford, Christine Riding, Martin Stiles, Sarah Victoria Turner and Hannah Williams. Finally, thanks to Paul Holberton and Laura Parker of Paul Holberton Publishing for their unwavering belief in this project and for producing the beautiful book that I had always hoped for; and the exhibition team at the Foundling Museum, Janette Bright, Stephanie Chapman, Alison Duke, Kathleen Palmer, and particularly Museum Director and chum, Caro Howell, without whom the exhibition and this publication would never have happened.

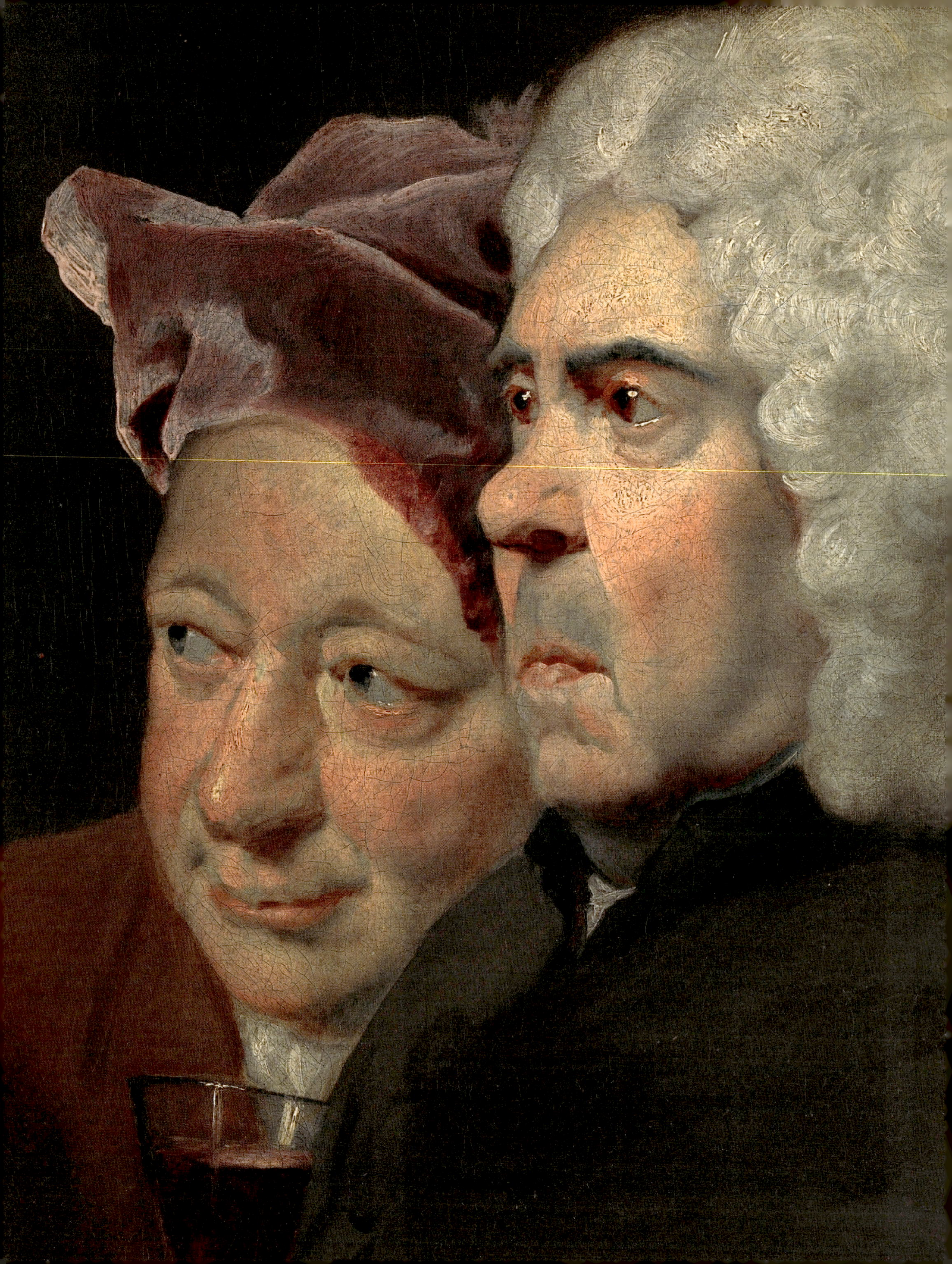

'MR. HIGHMORE'

On the morning of Friday 5 March 1762, the auctioneer Abraham Langford arrived at a house on Holborn Row, Lincoln's Inn Fields. At twelve o'clock prompt he would begin the sale of the 'GENUINE and ENTIRE COLLECTION of PICTURES OF Mr. JOSEPH HIGHMORE'.[1] The sixty-nine-year-old painter had decided to retire on the marriage of his only daughter the previous year. He was now preparing to leave his home and studio of almost thirty-seven years to live with Susanna and his son-in-law, the Reverend John Duncombe, in their house within the precincts of Canterbury Cathedral.[2] From the evidence of his documented output, it is clear that in reality Highmore had been in semi-retirement for most of the previous decade. One catalyst for this slowdown in his artistic activity may have been the untimely death of his beloved wife Susanna in 1750.

It is also the case that, in these same years, Highmore was developing new interests as an author.[3] After his formal retirement in 1762, writing and publishing became Highmore's chief intellectual occupation.[4] The essays and pamphlets he wrote in these years contain insights into his thoughts and opinions on subjects as wide-ranging as art theory and practice, theology and philosophy, and a broad selection of these observations has been introduced and discussed in the present study. However, the focus here is Highmore's practice as an artist and particularly the highly active and varied career he pursued during the 1740s, a decade which saw him diversify beyond his core activity, portraiture.

The contents of Highmore's studio sale in 1762 bears witness to this variety. The sale contained 79 lots covering 138 individual works, of which a majority were by Highmore himself. Unsurprisingly, a large proportion of these paintings were portraits, with all formats represented – from bust-lengths and 'kit-cats' to full-lengths, and from single figures to family groups. Among the portraits were seven royal images, mostly full-lengths, including a painting of King James II/VII after Sir Peter Lely and pictures of King George II and his son Frederick Louis, Prince of Wales with their consorts.[5] The aristocracy and gentry were represented by figures such as 'the Earl of Buckinghamshire'[6] and the six half-lengths of the family of Sir William Gordon of Invergordon, including Anne Dundas née Gordon, Lady Arniston, possibly a copy of the painting now at Arniston House, Midlothian.

Among the remaining portraits were thirteen images of 'celebrities' including kit-cats 'from memory' of Elizabeth and Maria Gunning, the famed Irish beauties who caused a sensation on their arrival in London in 1751.[7] A half-length painting by Highmore labelled as 'Maria, Countess of Coventry' is now at Waddesdon Manor, Buckinghamshire.[8] The portrait of Highmore's most unusual sitter was also included in the sale – 'the famous *Buckinger*' or Mathew Buchinger (1674–1740), a public entertainer from Germany who had been born with no hands or legs.[9] Buchinger toured England in the 1720s and early 1730s, and this portrait (untraced) is an earlier example of Highmore's interest in newsworthy personalities. Finally, there were portraits in the manner of eminent Flemish and Dutch seventeenth-century artists such as Sir Peter Paul Rubens and Rembrandt van Rijn.

In addition to portraiture, the sale contained eight history paintings by Highmore, both original

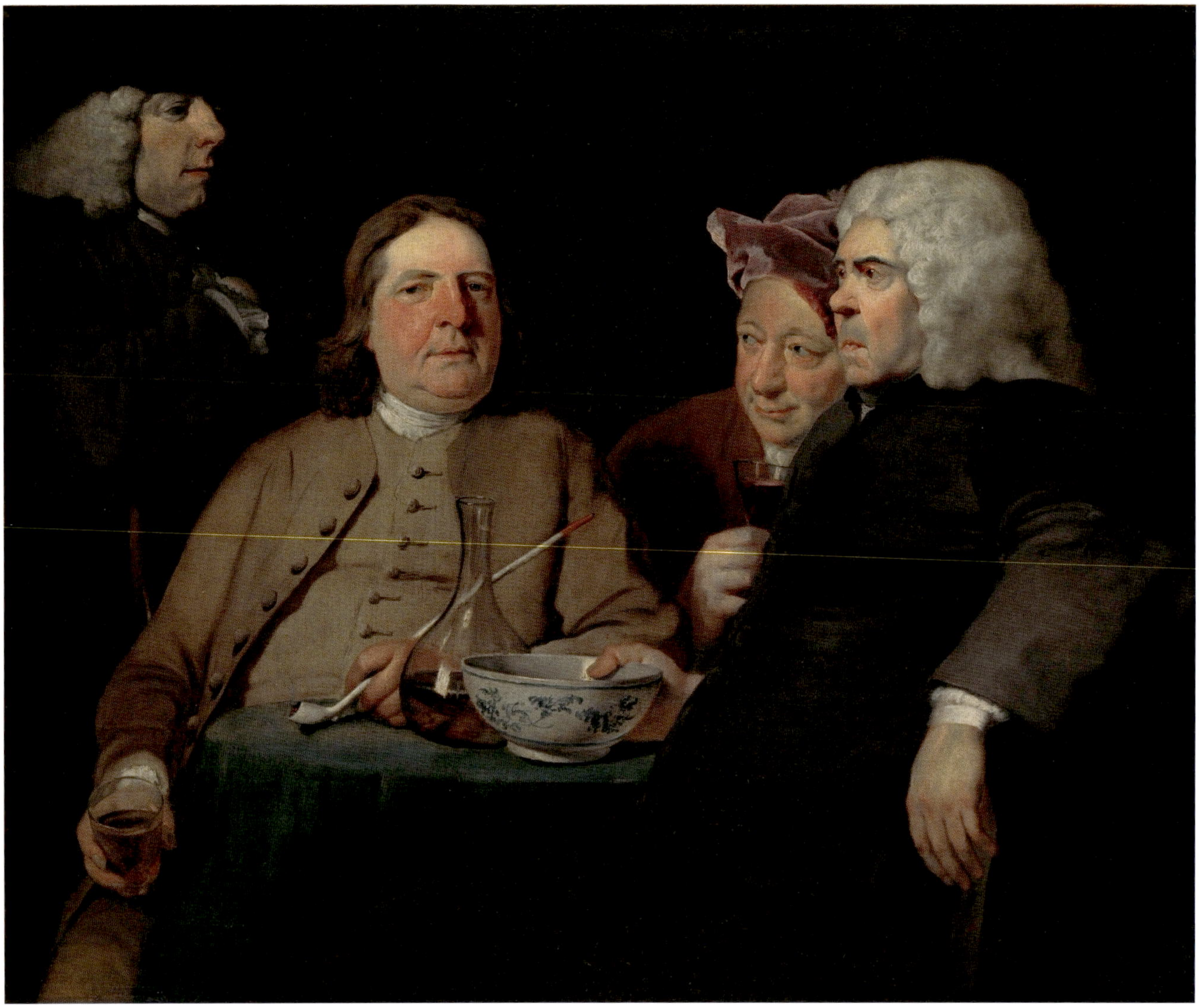

1 Joseph Highmore, *Mr Oldham and his Guests*, c.1735–45, oil on canvas, 105.5 x 129.5 cm, Tate

The portrait commemorates a supper held at Nathaniel Oldham's house in Ealing, where the affable and slightly eccentric host, a keen huntsman (standing left), arrived very late. Highmore, who painted at least two other portraits of his friend, is traditionally identified as the figure in the pink velvet cap.

canvases and copies after Flemish and Italian painters. One of his original works was a large canvas (untraced) representing a scene from the reign of King Richard III which had been displayed unfinished at the Society of Artists exhibition in 1760.[10] More traditional subjects included the biblical narratives 'The Wisemen's offering' and 'the Purification of the Virgin, its Companion'.[11] The subject-matter of fifteen of the paintings in the sale derived from the novels of Samuel Richardson (1689–1761).[12] Finally, there were examples of landscape and topographical painting, 'Two Landscapes', '2 Views of *Apsted Park*, and the Duke of *Bridgewater*'s Park and House' and '*Isleworth*'.[13]

Two centuries later, a visitor to the Joseph Highmore exhibition at Kenwood House in London would have gained some idea of the contents of the artist's house on that March day in 1762. The display brought together forty-two paintings, offering a modest survey of every decade from the 1720s to the 1760s.[14] The exhibits included the twelve paintings inspired by Samuel Richardson's *Pamela* (painted 1743–44), a version of a portrait of Frederick Louis, Prince of Wales, a self-portrait (see fig. 7), the portrait of his daughter (see fig. 9) and *Mr. Oldham and his Guests* (fig. 1). Prior to the Foundling Museum exhibition in 2017–18, this had been the only major monographic exhibition dedicated to Highmore's work and it was a key event for three reasons.

First, it drew public attention to an artist whose reputation had declined dramatically over the centuries, as the misattributions to Hogarth of both *The Angel of Mercy* and *Mr Oldham and his Guests* indicate. In fact, it is a decline that can be charted from within years of Highmore's death. In 1782 the second edition of Horace Walpole's influential *Anecdotes of Painting in England* was published.[15] It continued to be promoted as a 'digested' account from the extensive notebooks of the engraver and habitual chronicler of the early Georgian art world, George Vertue (1684–1756).[16] In reality, as we now know, it is a highly selective, partial and therefore deeply flawed assessment of the period concerned, which cheerfully ignores a majority of Vertue's observations and insights on the art and artists of his time. Walpole's derisively brief biographical entry on Highmore, which names only one example from the enormous range of the artist's output, alongside his two publications on perspective, is in dramatic contrast to the details provided in the *Memoirs* or obituary written by Highmore's son-in-law and published only two years before (*The Gentleman's Magazine*, April 1780).[17]

Walpole's subjectivity is exposed with his statement, 'Having dispatched the herd of our painters in oil, I reserved to a class by himself that great and original genius, Hogarth'.[18] Sixteen years on, in unison with Walpole, John Ireland declared in his *Hogarth Illustrated* (in excusing the artist's legendary tetchiness),

> If it should be thought that Hogarth, in the course of his narration, seems too tremblingly alive, and sometimes offended where offence was not meant, let it be recollected, that he must have felt superior to men whom the public preferred. To rank him with Kent, Jervas, Highmore, Hudson, Hayman, or any of that school of mannerists who figured in the different periods of his life, is classing a giant among pigmies.[19]

This negative assessment of Highmore, indeed of every artist of his generation excepting Hogarth, remained more or less intact until the mid twentieth century. Such an assessment completely ignores the impact of professional rivalry, fuelled by a steely competitiveness, on Hogarth's artistic development. Put another way, I would argue, Hogarth would never have become a great artist if he had been surrounded by artistic 'pigmies'. For Highmore, the Kenwood exhibition in 1963 signalled at the very least that a return to prominence was gradually occurring, after many decades – if not centuries – of condescension and obscurity.

Secondly, the exhibition was a tangible result of the independent scholarship of important twentieth-century figures working in British art, namely, John Scobell Armstrong, Charles Beard, J.W. Goodison, Charles Collins Baker, Frederick Antal and Ralph Edwards.[20] Collectively, their perceptive articles and reattributions created the environment within which Highmore could be considered a worthy subject not only for an exhibition but for serious academic study. This new scholarship included a doctoral thesis on the artist, Alison Shepherd Lewis's *Joseph Highmore: an eighteenth-century English portrait painter* 1692–1780 (1975, reprinted 1976), the first attempt at a full biography and survey of the artist's work.[21]

Thirdly, the exhibition led to an extraordinary discovery. During his speech at the opening event, Highmore's descendant Sir Anthony Highmore King produced from his pocket Highmore's journal, written during his trip to Paris in 1734.[22] Until that moment, scholars of British art had been unaware of the existence of this document, the single most important

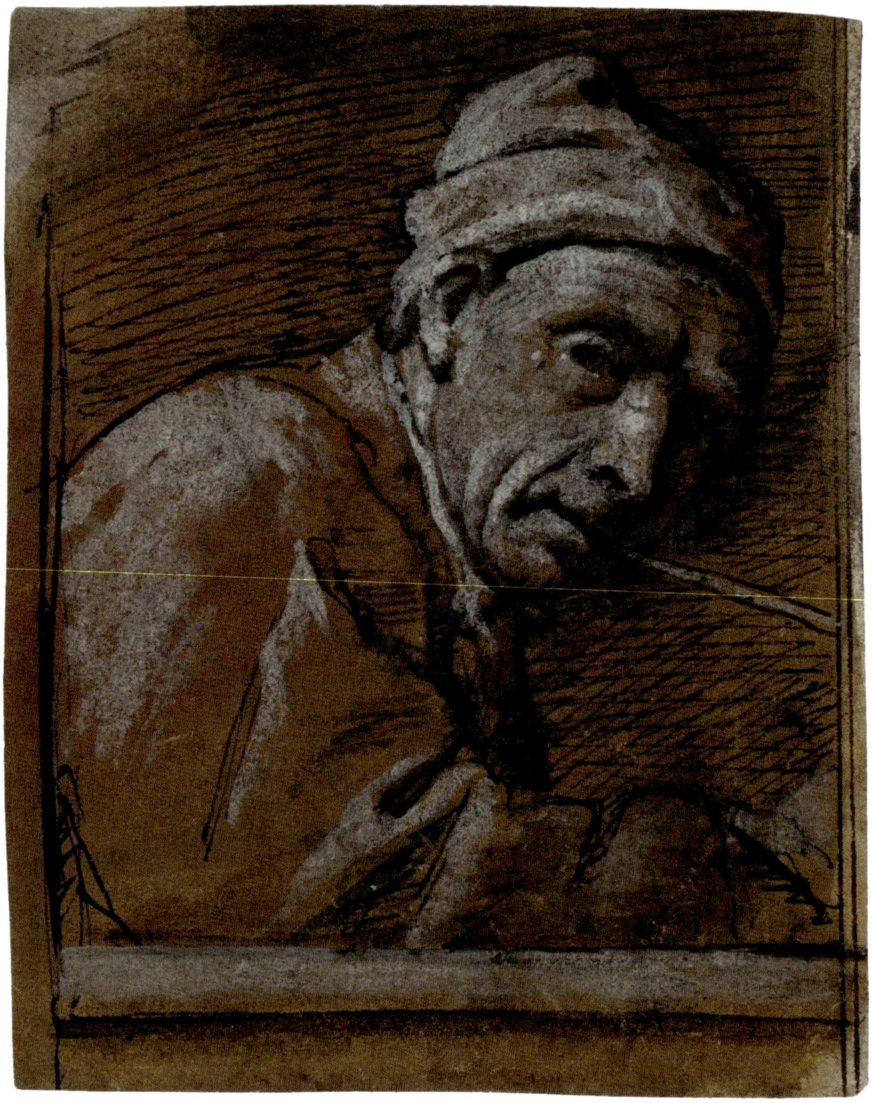

2 Joseph Highmore, *Portrait of a man in a cap*, date not known, graphite, ink and watercolour on paper, 108 x 89 mm, Tate

This is likely to be a self-portrait and dateable to the same period as *Mr Oldham and his Guests* (fig. 1).

manuscript in Highmore's hand and a rare example of an English artist's travel journal from the early Georgian period.[23] In 1986 a collection of drawings and archive material – described as 'The Highmore Family Gift' – was donated to the Tate Gallery, in Sir Anthony's honour, by his heirs.[24] The collection in its entirety, which includes the Paris journal, has not been researched, as yet, in any great detail (figs. 2 and 3). This current study, alongside the MA dissertation and doctoral thesis which underpin it, has benefitted immensely from this extremely rich cache of material.

Turning to later scholarship, Elizabeth Einberg's exhibition publication *Manners & Morals: Hogarth and British Painting 1700–1760* (1986) and her catalogue, written with Judy Egerton, of the Tate Gallery's early

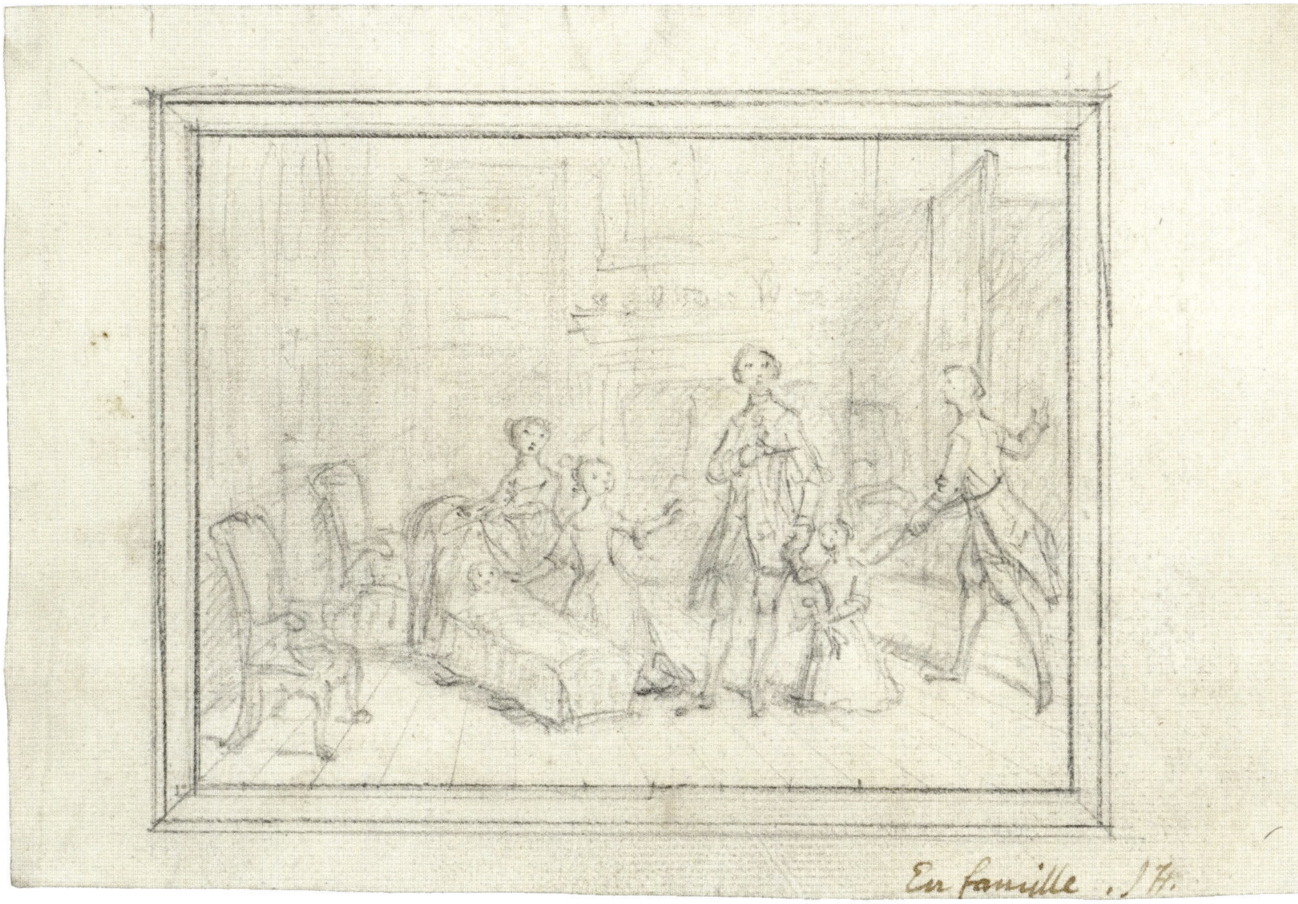

3 Joseph Highmore, *Family group of six persons in a room*, date not known, graphite on paper, 127 x 192 mm, Tate

The note in brown ink reads *En famille* with the monogram *J H*. The inscriptions are believed to be by Joseph Highmore's grandson, Anthony (1758–1829), in which case this is a sketch by Highmore for a portrait of his son, also Anthony (1718–1799), and grandchildren. Anthony and his wife Anna Maria were married in 1740 and had fifteen children, only two of whom, Anthony and Sarah, survived him.

Georgian works of art, *The Age of Hogarth: British Painters born 1675–1709* (1988) remained, until recently, the most extensive published texts on individual works by Highmore: to these can now be added five further articles and the present study.[25]

The art world in the 'Age of Hogarth', whose engine was London, was as dynamic, innovative, sophisticated and cosmopolitan as the metropolis itself. Focusing on one artist, even if that artist is William Hogarth, cannot adequately reflect the city and population in all its richness and variety, let alone, more broadly, the early Georgian period in Great Britain and Ireland. A study of the career of Joseph Highmore, alongside his contemporaries Hogarth, Thomas Hudson, Francis Hayman and Charles Jervas among many others, adds a necessary depth and breadth to our appreciation and understanding of this vibrant world.

In many ways, the Foundling Hospital – the institution and its people – was early Georgian society in little. After all it was a place where the richest and poorest, the powerful and the disenfranchised, the most cosseted and the most vulnerable came together, no matter how fleetingly. And, through countless tales of misery and hope, it represented the very best and the very worst of human nature.

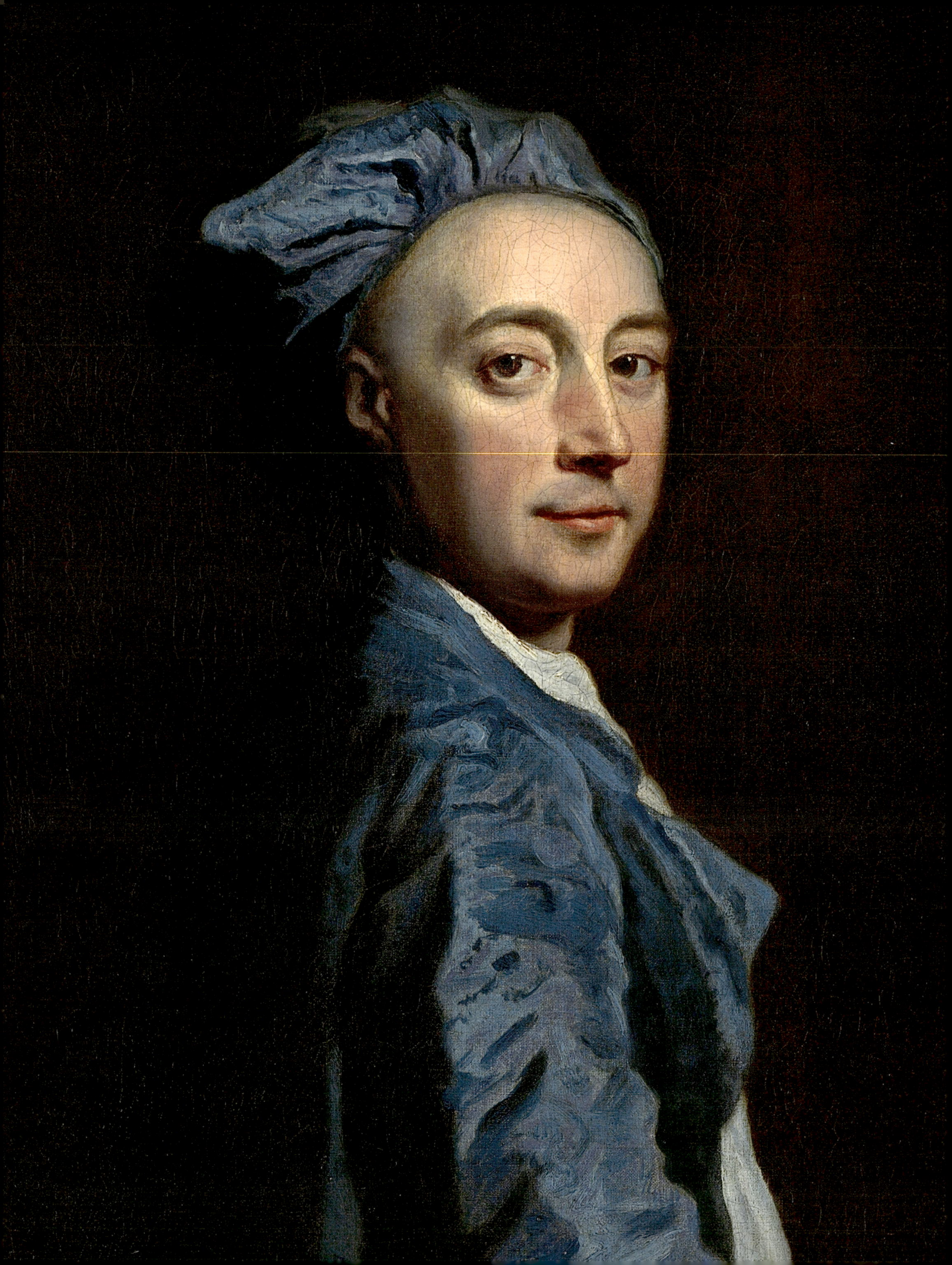

'AN INGENIOUS YOUNG PAINTER'

Joseph Highmore was born in Thames Street in the City of London parish of St James Garlickhithe on 13 June 1692, the third son of Edward, a coal merchant.[1] Highmore's father appears to have had a thriving business. One advertisement in the *Daily Courant* 26 November 1720 announced, 'There is a considerable Quantity of Cannel Coal from Sir Roger Bradshaigh's Pitts in Lancashire brought to Town, and are to be sold at Mr. Highmore's Wharf at Trigg-Stairs in Thames-Street'.[2] Young Joseph attended the nearby City of London 'Free Grammar' School, Merchant Taylors' in Suffolk Lane from 1701/02–04.[3] From the foundation of the school in 1561, it was a requirement that all students on entering should be able to read and write. Classical learning in Latin and Greek was a core element of the curriculum and, in addition, Highmore may have been taught Hebrew.[4]

More important still was the observance of Protestant Christianity.[5] As late as the early nineteenth century the scholars were still required, as set out in the founding statutes, 'thrice in the day, kneeling on their knees, they shall say the prayers appointed with due tract and pawsing'.[6] The Reverend Wilson later observed that it was such 'useful learning' that had 'so remarkably enlightened the middle ranks of the English nation'.[7] The poet Edmund Spenser (c.1552–1599) and playwright Ben Jonson (1572–1637) had both attended the school, and among Highmore's contemporaries were future City bankers, members of the Royal Society and archbishops.[8]

Clearly Merchant Taylors' encouraged a strong work ethic, personal restraint, and a sense of social status among the professional 'middling sort'.

George Vertue observed that Highmore had 'many good qualifications absolutely necessary towards cultivating the theory of the Art', which he lists as a 'good education' accompanied by 'a very sober conduct' and 'a resolute mind to overcome the dificulties [sic]'. The mention of difficulties could relate to family pressure to follow a legal career. But from Vertue's short description we learn that the young Highmore was intelligent, dedicated and determined. The seven years that he was associated with the law, during his clerkship to a City attorney, provided him with what we would now call social skills and 'polish', as Vertue, in one of his most pointedly revealing comments concerning the painter's manner, makes clear: 'the Natural practice of the Law gives most men. a good Voluble speech with a Stedfast assurance. of which he has benefitted in that particular. & turns it well to his advantage, needing not that as many ingenious men do'.[9] Vertue hints that Highmore had the type of easy charm, confidence and eloquence that might gain him *entrée* to social circles, and therefore commissions, that otherwise would have been beyond his reach.

Regarding artistic training, Vertue, who in 1723 described Highmore as 'an ingenious young painter', noted that prior to his membership of the Great Queen Street Academy (from 1713, then under the governorship of Britain's leading portrait-painter Sir Godfrey Kneller [1646–1723]) Highmore 'made great improvements by practice & observation haveing no Master to teach him regularly'.[10] The *Memoirs* of 1780 offer additional information on this subject:

> Having such an early and strong inclination to painting, that he could think of nothing else with pleasure, his father endeavoured to gratify him in a proposal to his uncle, who was serjeant-painter to King William, and with whom Mr. (afterwards, Sir James) Thornhill had served his apprenticeship. But this was afterwards for good reasons declined.[11]

In the event, Highmore may not have received any training and guidance from his uncle, despite the natural assumption that Thomas Highmore would have assisted a close relative to enter his profession at the behest of his own brother.[12] As the *Memoirs* confirm, Thomas had a studio and apprentices and therefore could have accommodated his nephew. More pertinent still, Thomas Highmore's apprentices had included the most significant English-born artist of the early eighteenth century, the history painter James Thornhill (1675/76–1734).[13] As Serjeant-painter, Thomas had direct connection to the royal family and court and therefore important channels of patronage. All of which would have been extremely useful to his young nephew, as it had proved for Thornhill his cousin by marriage.[14]

Although generally reliable, Vertue is incorrect in his statement that Highmore 'left the law to study painting'.[15] In fact Highmore had continued with both, pursuing his art studies in his spare time, until he was finally freed from his seven-year clerkship. As the *Memoirs* state, this clerkship was

> so much against his own declared inclination, that in about three years he began to form resolutions of indulging his natural disposition to his favourite art, having continually employed his leisure hours designing, and in the study of geometry, perspective, architecture, and anatomy, but without any instructors except books.[16]

This establishes the thoroughness of Highmore's self-directed study. Meanwhile, the statement that he had no 'instructors except books' might, at first glance, confirm a lack of formal or informal art teaching. The *Memoirs* go on to state that

> He had afterwards an opportunity of improving himself in anatomy, by attending the lectures of Mr. Cheselden, besides entering himself at the Painter's Academy in Great Queen-street, where he drew 10 years, and had the honour to be particularly noticed by Sir Godfrey Kneller, who distinguished him by the name of *the Young Lawyer*.[17]

Highmore's attendance at the anatomy classes of the celebrated surgeon William Cheselden (1688–1752) resulted in two illustrations for the second edition of Cheselden's *The Anatomy of the Human Body* (London, 1722), Plates XII and XIII. Both, according to the *Memoirs*, were engraved from 'drawings from the real subjects at the time of dissection'.[18] Highmore's interest in anatomy and attendance at dissections reveal a general inquisitiveness, as well as a diligence in developing the necessary skills and knowledge for a career in art.

Nonetheless, Kneller's nickname for Highmore, 'the young lawyer', suggests that, during his early years at this artist-led and informal drawing academy, Highmore was known for his legal associations rather than for any obvious artistic ambition or potential. It suggests that he maintained a level of secrecy about his intentions during those years. After all, geometry, perspective and architecture were all areas fit for gentlemanly study as well as professional training. Highmore's interest in geometry and particularly perspective remained with him throughout his career and retirement, resulting, as mentioned earlier, in the production of two publications.[19] That Highmore was acknowledged as something of an authority on the subject is suggested by the presence of *The Practice of Perspective, on the Principles of Dr. Brook Taylor* (London, 1763) in the library of one J.M.W. Turner (1775–1851), who was, between 1807 and 1837, Professor of Perspective at the Royal Academy of Arts.[20]

Vertue's comment, that Highmore 'turn'd his genius to portrait painting', is an important one. The phrase follows the observation that he 'came into the Accademy drew several years there fell into acquaintance with most of the ingenious masters & young students',[21] which suggests that in discussion with, as well as observing, the artists of the academy,

Highmore made a conscious decision to become a painter of portraits rather than history or landscape. Crucially, like many of his peers, Highmore chose to focus on the genre within British art practice that provided most opportunity for regular employment, rather than the genre that was considered, by tradition, the greatest in the hierarchy of painting. As we shall see, Highmore would focus on portraiture for twenty-five years before attempting a public career in history painting.

Vertue's description of Highmore as having 'a very sober conduct' hints at someone with a character that was clear-headed, resolute and sensible, and perhaps unsentimental regarding the stark realities of the market for contemporary art – as his choice of focus indicates. Thomas Highmore, Thornhill and Kneller can all be described as mentors during his early training and career. Yet it is the Dutch artist Hendrik van der Straaten (c.1665–1722) who seems to have been the original trigger for Highmore's interest in painting. It can also be argued that it was Van der Straaten who impressed upon the young Highmore an understanding of painting as a process, a profession and, on a very basic level, an income generator.

Van der Straaten lived in Wylde Street near Drury Lane and was humorously described by the *London Literary Gazette* over a century later as 'decorator-general to all the taverns and tea-gardens within the bills of mortality'.[22] Highmore, on the other hand, described him as 'perhaps the most expeditious painter that ever lived'.[23] According to Highmore, Van der Straaten painted landscapes on one long canvas, almost in the manner of theatre scenery, which he then cut up and sold in 'pieces' – art that was literally being produced and sold by the yard. Highmore observed in 1764 that 'he had something like genius and taste, and painted much in the manner of Francisque [possibly the Flemish landscape painter Francisque Millet (1642–1679)], and did all that could be done in the time he allowed himself'.[24] There is admiration in this comment, in part directed at Van der Straaten's awareness of his artistic limitations and, more importantly, his knowledge of his market. The observation that Van der Straaten 'did all that could be done in the time he allowed himself' suggests a pragmatic professional, who had reconciled artistic integrity with the daily grind of a commercial art practice. Highmore concludes, 'I remember the man: he was the first I ever saw paint, and I may perhaps be partial to him on that account, having had great pleasure, when young, in visiting him'.[25]

By 1715, then, Highmore would have experienced a solid, gentlemanly education, gaining a knowledge in at least Latin and Greek, which was enhanced by focused self-directed study.[26] He had benefitted immensely from his attendance at the Great Queen Street Academy, after possibly gaining some advice and rudimentary training from his uncle. Even so, he was largely a self-taught artist, who had shown great perseverance, determination and not a little guile in pursuit of his artistic ambitions. He also possessed the insider knowledge, connections and skills of a City-based professional. Highmore's formation and training are particular. They influenced his painting practice and his vision and identity as an artist.

'GOOD EMPLOY AMONGST THE CITIZENS'

Highmore completed his articles in June 1714 and eight months later he publicly launched his portrait-painting practice. As the *Memoirs* record, 'On June 13, 1714 [Highmore's birthday, he was twenty-two years old] his clerkship expired; on March 26, 1715, he began painting as a profession, and settled in the city'.[27] Presumably Highmore had gained sufficient encouragement and therefore artistic confidence to make such a bold, even audacious move, despite his lack of regular formal training and having been a member of Kneller's academy for only two years. It certainly removed any potential for a career in law, for the foreseeable future at least. In the meantime, Highmore continued attending the academy, which from about 1718 was under the governorship of James Thornhill, and then went on to subscribe to a new artist academy in St Martin's Lane, established in 1720 by his precocious contemporary John Vanderbank (1694–1739) and the veteran French-born history painter

Louis Chéron (1660–1725).[28] It is worth stressing the international nature of the directors, teachers and membership of these early London art academies. They were forums for debate on issues of art theory as well as practice, alongside other subjects of intellectual and practical relevance to art, including natural philosophy, medicine, history and literature.[29]

In his 1726 account, Vertue observes that Highmore had established his practice in the City rather than London's expanding West End, where 'he [had] good employ. amongst the Citizens'. Crucially, Highmore was a native of this particular area of London – now nicknamed 'the Square Mile' – and his local schooling and clerkship would have provided vital contacts and future clients. The six known commissioned portraits prior to 1723 testify that it was the City-based merchants – including Thomas Hollis (1659–1731), benefactor of Harvard College, Massachusetts – scholars and non-conformist churchmen that offered a natural, regular and lucrative client base for the young artist.[30] Indeed, through the Hollis commission, Highmore achieved some fame as far afield as the American colonies at a very early stage in his career. In a letter to Harvard's president, John Leverett, dated 26 September 1722, Hollis wrote, regarding the delivery of his portrait: 'The painter thinks that the Picture being nailed up a long voyage may [be] a little flatt the paint it being so newly finished, but after it has been some time hung up in your Hall the airs may recover its proper colour'.[31] It was destroyed by fire in 1764, but is known through the mezzotint produced in Boston by Peter Pelham.[32]

Through these contacts, Highmore quickly achieved reputational and financial success, so much so that he was able to marry Susanna Hiller, a yeoman farmer's daughter from Surrey, on 28 May 1716.[33] In 1718 their first child, Anthony, was born.[34]

In regard to portrait style and composition, Vertue noted in 1723 that Highmore was 'very correct & just in his representations & imitations of nature'.[35] Vertue continues that Highmore produced such likenesses 'with a free masterly manner his pencil free & bold', 'his colours natural & lively', indicating a confidence with the mechanics of painting, whether in design or the application of paint to canvas, and some fluidity and flair in the result. Having described the 'human' elements of portraiture, Vertue moved on to the costume: 'his draperys the habits as worn very natural'. In Vertue's opinion, Highmore attempted and succeeded in presenting nothing beyond what was there before him – an honest, accurate and skilful replication of his subject. One of the earliest extant portraits by Highmore is of the ivory carver David Le Marchand (c.1723; fig. 4), which supports Vertue's basic assessment of the painter's portrait style at this time. And yet, through the dramatic pose and bold lighting, the portrait hints at a shift in ambition and inventiveness. The long illness of Sir Godfrey Kneller, who was also Principal Painter to the King, and his subsequent death in October 1723 may have acted as a spur to Highmore, as well as his fellow portrait-painters, to raise his game.[36]

Vertue concluded his 1726 account of Highmore's career by declaring that 'he is lately removd to Lincolns Inn fields'.[37] The timing of the artist's relocation west to a more fashionable area of the capital, just beyond the confines of the City, is confirmed in the *Memoirs* as March 1724.[38] Within six months of the death of Kneller, therefore, Highmore had moved his small family, his studio and his practice away from the site and patronage base of his early career. Elaborating upon Vertue's statement, the *Memoirs* observe that 'His reputation and business increasing, he took a more conspicuous station, by removing to a house in Lincoln's Inn Fields'.[39] Soon after moving to their new home, Joseph and Susanna's second child, Susanna, was born (1725).

The phrase 'a more conspicuous station' confirms that Highmore's intention in moving was, at least in part, to display his current success and status, while laying the ground for a new kind of career path. Given the local presence of portraitists such as Jonathan Richardson (1667–1745) and Bartholomew Dandridge (1691–c.1754), Highmore's relocation to Lincoln's Inn Fields signalled a conscious move into the heart of the artist community then centred around Great Queen Street.

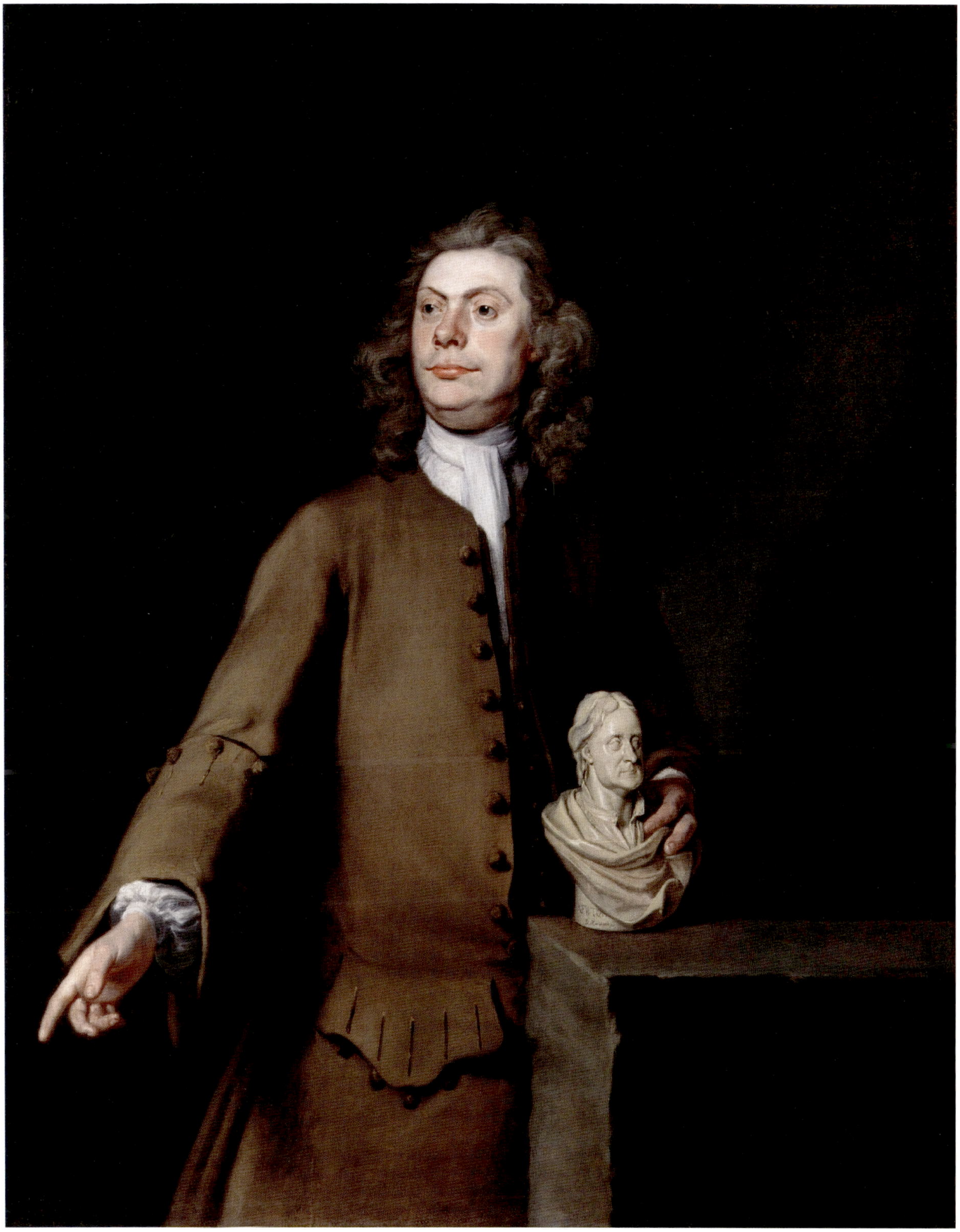

4 Joseph Highmore, *David Le Marchand*, c.1723,
oil on canvas, 124 x 99.7 cm, National Portrait Gallery, London

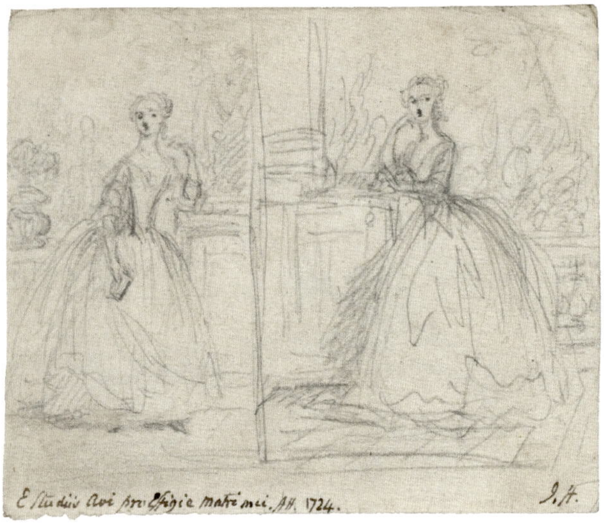

5 Joseph Highmore, *Two studies for a female full-length*, c.1740, graphite on paper, 143 x 172 mm, Tate

The inscription reads *E Studiis Avi pro Effigie Matri mei. AH. 1724. J.H.* It is believed that the inscriptions are by Joseph Highmore's grandson and therefore the sitter is Anthony's mother, and the artist's daughter-in-law, Anna Maria née Ellis. However, the inscriber could be Joseph Highmore's son and the sitter, therefore, the artist's wife Susanna, which would tally with the given date of 1724.

Highmore's new residence, which he maintained until he retired in 1762, was located on the north side of the square, a few houses east from Richardson's home and studio. While Highmore resided here, Richardson was to vacate this house in favour of his pupil and son-in-law Thomas Hudson, who in turn housed his pupil, Joshua Reynolds, in the early 1740s.[40] Therefore the area continued to be an important centre for artists throughout Highmore's residency. It was a convenient and suitably genteel location for clients, potential clients and impromptu visitors, and one that was more appropriate for an ambitious portrait-painter than the parish of St Swithin's. However, the fact that Lincoln's Inn Fields sits between the City and the West End allowed Highmore to attract potential clients residing in London's new developments to the west while maintaining close proximity to his legal contacts at the Inns of Court – particularly Lincoln's Inn – and to his established clientele in the City.

The house that Highmore leased no longer exists, but an advertisement in the *General Advertiser* from 1749, regarding the sale of the plot which included Highmore's residence, describes a substantial property: 'No. 6, Four Rooms on a Floor, with a Coach-House and Stables, let to Mr. Highmore, by Mistake at 60 l. worth 90 1. a Year'.[41] That Highmore managed to rent the property for two thirds of its actual value might be an indication of that suave legal manner in action. Houses in Lincoln's Inn Fields usually have three full floors (ground to second), a garret floor above and kitchens in the basement. With four rooms per floor – potentially two large rooms at the front, a third set behind next to the stairwell, with a closet-room leading off it – this was certainly a comfortable family home, studio and exhibiting space. The rear of the house would have faced north (a consideration for maximum and even light) but, as potentially larger rooms with a greater number of windows were located at the front, overlooking the square, Highmore's painting room may have been located on this side of the building.

A hint as to how the house might have been arranged can be gleaned from Highmore's group portrait of his family (currently dated c.1732; fig. 6). This is likely to show the two rooms on the first floor at the front, as indicated by the window to the immediate left and, through the open door, by what appears to be light from another window in the same location in the room beyond. The raised and fielded panels of the wainscot panelling indicate that this is a high-level room within the hierarchy of the interior decoration (therefore on the 'principal' or first floor) but the interior is modestly furnished: no textiles can be seen at the window casement or seat, the olive or 'drab' painted panelling is hung with a single over-door canvas (probably a landscape), the furniture consists of one chair upholstered in an ochre silk damask, a small round walnut table and a turkey rug. There is, as yet, no trace of the sizable collection of paintings that we know Highmore stored and displayed at this house, including full-length canvases. The room just visible beyond the open door may be a library, as there is a hint of the cross

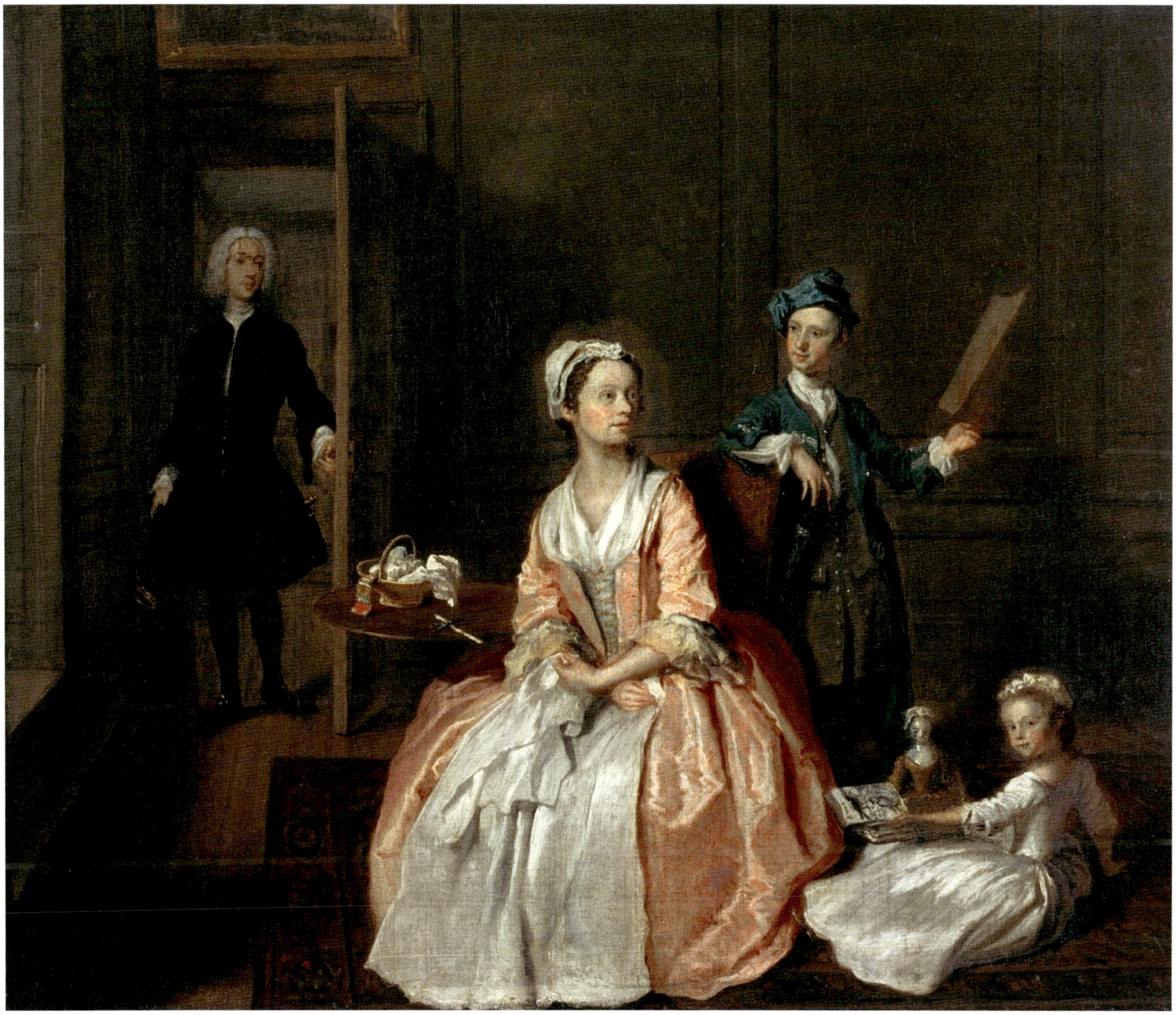

6 Joseph Highmore, *The Artist and his Family*, c.1732, oil on canvas, 64.7 x 77.5 cm, private collection

bars of shelving and the spines of large books on the visible wall.

Anthony, to the right, is dressed as a miniature version of his father, as seen in Highmore's self-portrait (fig. 7), with his distinctive Prussian-blue house cap and coat with silver lacing, a red pencil held nonchalantly in one hand and a drawing raised aloft in the other. Even at this young age, Anthony is presented as a gentleman artist at his leisure. Susanna is holding a book opened to illustrations of birds, as if she has been interrupted reading aloud to the doll sitting beside her. Meanwhile her mother, dressed in a rich coral-pink silk robe, pauses in her needlework.

Over a decade later, Highmore painted his daughter (fig. 9) with her pet cats and parrot, holding up one miniature from a selection of coloured drawings lying on the table before her – some of which, the doll cut-outs for example, can be identified as those now in the

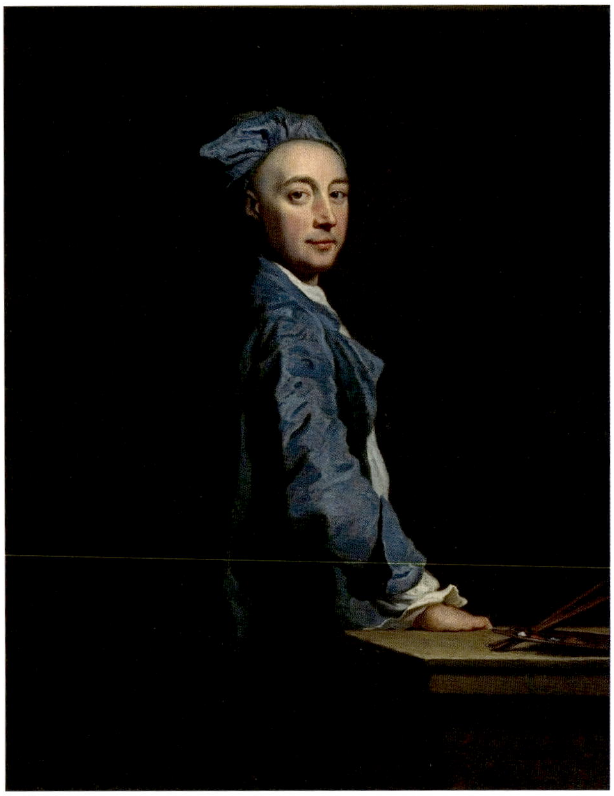

7 Joseph Highmore, *Self-portrait*, c.1745–47, oil on canvas, 126.4 x 101 cm, National Gallery of Victoria, Melbourne, Felton Bequest, 1947 (1760-4)

Given Highmore's relative youth, this self-portrait is datable to the late 1720s/early 1730s.

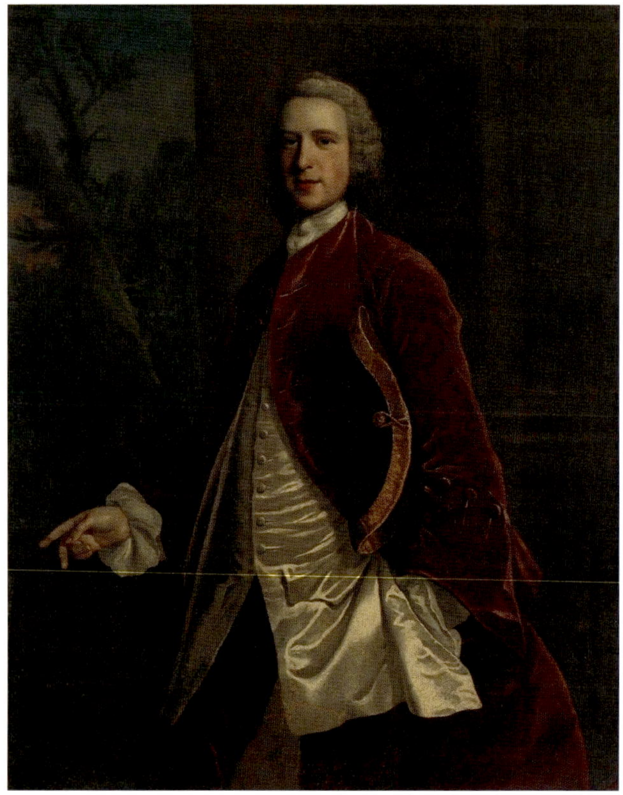

8 Joseph Highmore, *Anthony Highmore*, c.1745–47, oil on canvas, 126.4 x 101 cm, National Gallery of Victoria, Melbourne, Felton Bequest, 1947 (1759-4)

Highmore Family Gift (figs. 9 and 10). Susanna was a highly intelligent and educated young woman, fluent in French and Italian, yet with no aspirations to an artistic career, unlike her brother, beyond a modest reputation as a book illustrator. Her leisured existence is wittily set out in a letter from her friend the author and translator Elizabeth Carter (1717–1806), dated 1756:

> And so you are an arrant Frequenter of plays & operas, & leave poor Abbe du Boz to moulder o[n] his Shelf ... you will be mighty glad to have recourse to his Company in a few weeks when plays and operas will be no more, & you will be reduced to the lamentable Amusement of Wandering in Solitary Contemplation round the Basin in Lincolns Inn Fields.[42]

In addition to the Abbé Jean-Baptiste Du Bos (1670–1742), author of *Réflexions critiques sur la poésie et sur la peinture* (first published 1719), Elizabeth also refers to Susanna reading 'Boileau' (the critic and poet Nicolas Boileau-Despréaux, 1636–1711), the poet and librettist Pietro Metastasio (1698–1782; W.A. Mozart later set Metastasio's *La clemenza di Tito*), 'Boccalini' (probably the sixteenth-century satirist Traiano Boccalini) and Ludovico Ariosto's *Orlando Furioso* (first complete version published 1532). There are drawings by Susanna illustrating several scenes from Ariosto in the Highmore Family Gift.[43] Her relatively late marriage, aged thirty-six, suggests a resistance to surrendering her happy life as a 'blue stocking' while, after her mother's death, managing the Highmore household.

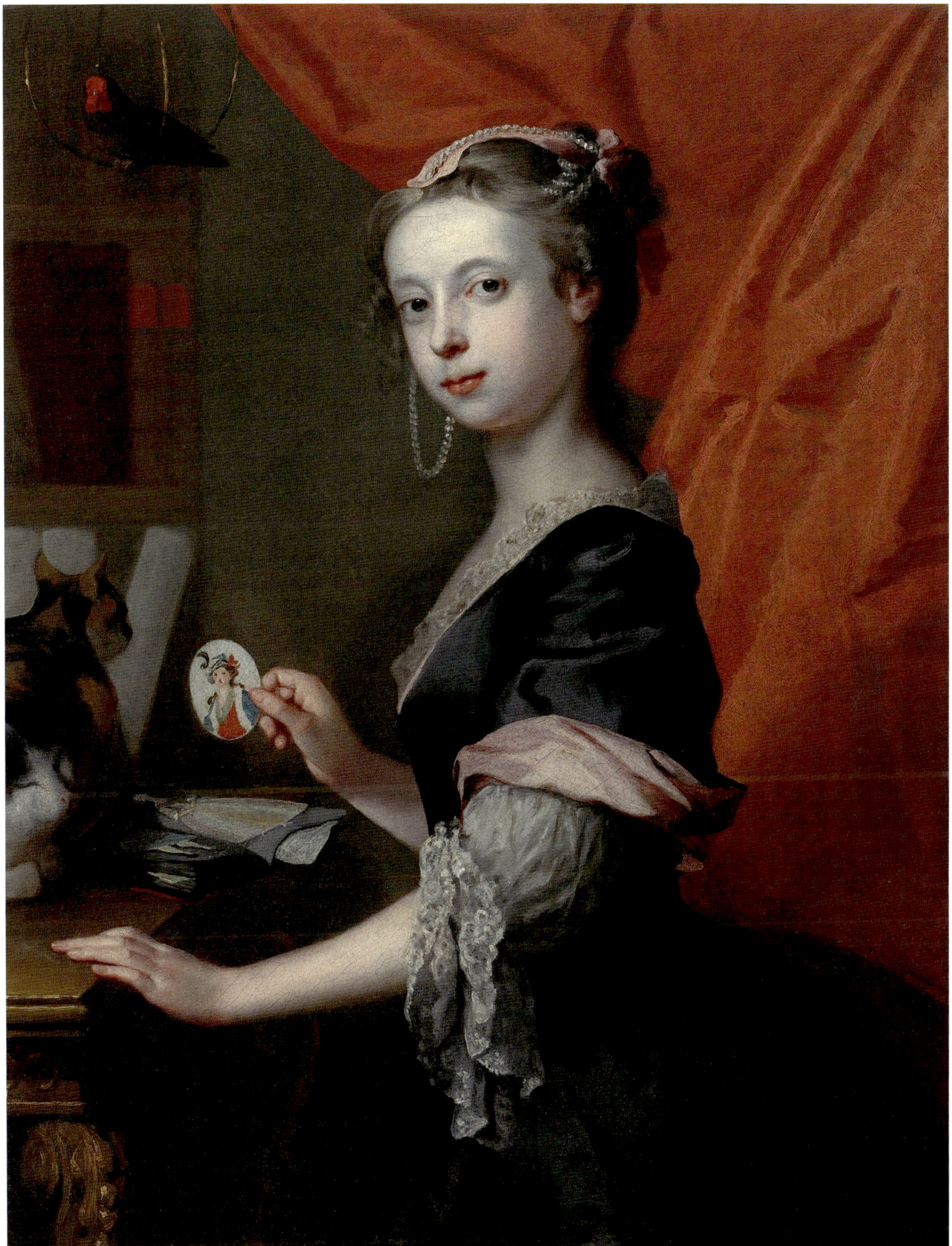

9 Joseph Highmore, *Susanna Highmore*, c.1740–45, oil on canvas, 91.5 x 71.1 cm, National Gallery of Victoria, Melbourne, Felton Bequest, 1947 (1761–4)

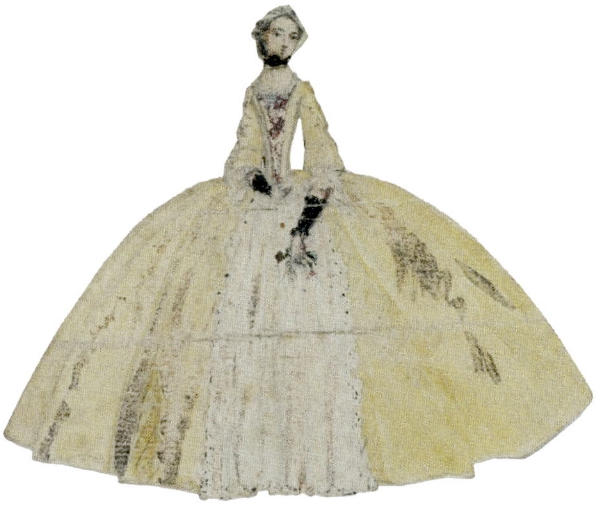

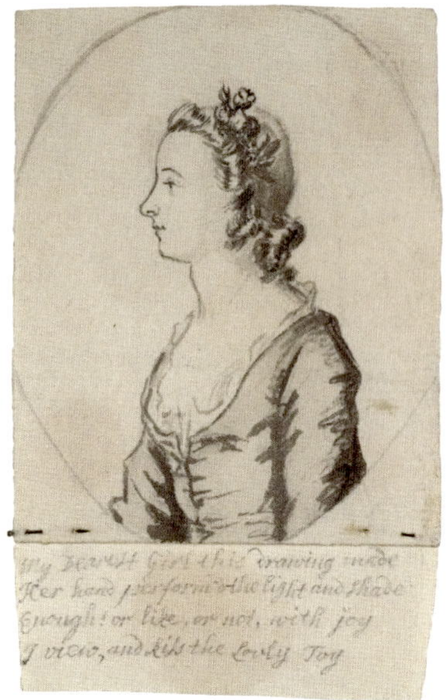

10 Susanna Duncombe née Highmore, Cut-out doll of a *Lady in Yellow*, date not known, graphite, watercolour and gouache on paper, 110 x 135 mm, Tate

11 Susanna Duncombe née Highmore, *Portrait of a young girl in profile to the left, within a drawn oval*, date not known, graphite and watercolour on paper, 93 x 76 mm, Tate

The text, in Joseph Highmore's handwriting, reads: *My Dearest Girl this drawing made / Her hand perform'd the light and shade / Enough : or like, or not, with joy / I view, and kiss the Lovly Toy*. When compared with Highmore's portrait of his wife and children (fig. 15), a strong contender for the sitter of Susanna's sketch is her mother. Highmore's affectionate poem, directed towards both artist and sitter, supports this identification.

'A MORE CONSPICUOUS STATION'

The move, in 1724, to Lincoln's Inn Fields also coincided with Highmore's membership of the Freemasons. As his stated aim at this time was to be 'more conspicuous', this decision is unlikely to have been taken separately from its potential impact on his professional life and aspirations.[44] His selection of masonic lodge is the key. In 1725 Highmore is listed as a member of the Swan Lodge on East Street, Greenwich, some six miles away from Lincoln's Inn Fields and on the south side of the River Thames.[45] The lodge had been constituted on 24 December 1723, offering the possibility that he was a founding member while living in St Swithin's parish.[46] Highmore's seemingly eccentric decision to join a lodge so distant from his home is revealed as a potentially canny career move when the master of the Swan Lodge is revealed to be none other than Sir James Thornhill, who was then completing the hall (later named the Painted Hall) of the Royal Naval Hospital at Greenwich.[47] As has been noted, Thornhill and Highmore were distant relatives by marriage. Further, Thornhill had been the beneficiary both of Thomas Highmore's training and of his vacant court position. Clearly Highmore hoped that such regular and intimate contact with an influential artist-relative might finally pay dividends. He may have expected a specific commission at Greenwich or else access to court or royal patronage more generally. This slightly disgruntled comment from Highmore, regarding the portraits of King George I and his family within the hall, does suggest lingering professional pique: 'I say nothing of the Royal Family at the upper end of that very Hall, but that it is to be lamented he was obliged to perform what he was not properly qualified to undertake, and yet could not decline'.[48]

Around this time Highmore produced a small portrait etching of Thornhill in profile with the inscription *J. Highmore pinx. & fecit 1723*.[49] Later, in 1732, Highmore produced a second portrait of Thornhill, this time in oils, which was engraved by John Faber in the same year (fig. 12). The original is untraced, but the print was itself a masonic collaboration, as the portrait-subject, the painter and the engraver were all freemasons. On Thornhill's retirement from the role of Serjeant-painter in the same year as the mezzotint, Highmore may have had his sights on this position in emulation of his uncle, and hoped that Thornhill would recommend him as his successor. In the event, that honour went to Thornhill's son John and then later to his son-in-law, William Hogarth.

Highmore was not unusual in his membership of the freemasons. Hogarth, Hudson, Samuel Scott (1702–1772) and Louis-François Roubiliac (1702/05–1762), among others, were also artist members.[50] However, he was certainly, alongside Thornhill, the most active and high-ranking of such artist-masons, as the following announcement in the *Evening Journal* on 28 December 1727 confirms:

> Yesterday being St. John's Day, the ancient Society of Free and Accepted MASONS, held their annual grand Meeting at Mercer's-Hall, and chose the following Officers for the next Year, viz The Lord Colerane Grand Master, Alexander Chocke, Esq; Deputy Grand Master, Nathaniel Blackerby, Esq; and Joseph Highmore, Grand Wardens.[51]

As a Grand Warden, Highmore was one of the four most important officers in the Grand Lodge – the governing body of English freemasonry – which had been formed from four Westminster lodges in 1717.[52] In the few years since he had joined, Highmore had evidently made rapid progress, moving from apprentice to fellow and finally to master mason. As the foremost portrait-painter mason of the 1720s Highmore was a natural choice to paint the first Grand Master of the Grand Lodge, Anthony Sayer (1672?–1742).[53] This work is now lost. A mezzotint after the portrait was produced by John Faber in 1742, the year of Sayer's death, another masonic collaboration.

The aristocratic leadership and membership of the freemasons was clearly an attraction for the aspirant 'lower orders' in joining the fraternity. On a purely practical level, freemasonry was an arena in which artists could advance their status and client base. This was due to the freedom allowed within the lodges and the Grand Lodge to associate with members from the aristocracy and gentry, without the hindrance of normal social protocols. Yet Highmore's active membership of the society and particularly his high rank indicates that his interest was more than professionally opportunistic. As a thoughtful and inquisitive man, Highmore may have been intrigued by the more 'spiritual' and esoteric qualities of masonic understanding and ceremony. However, Highmore's intimate association with freemasonry is not mentioned in the *Memoirs*. It can be presumed that, initially at least, his membership was a combination of pragmatism and the beguiling sense of belonging to and advancing within a powerful, mutually supportive fraternity.

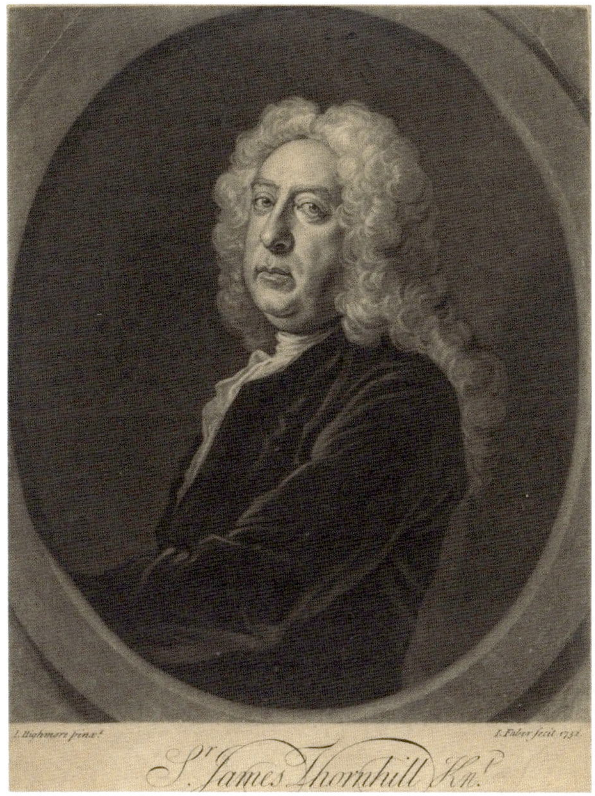

12 John Faber the Younger after Joseph Highmore, *Sir James Thornhill*, 1732, mezzotint, 328 x 252 mm, Yale Center for British Art, Paul Mellon Collection

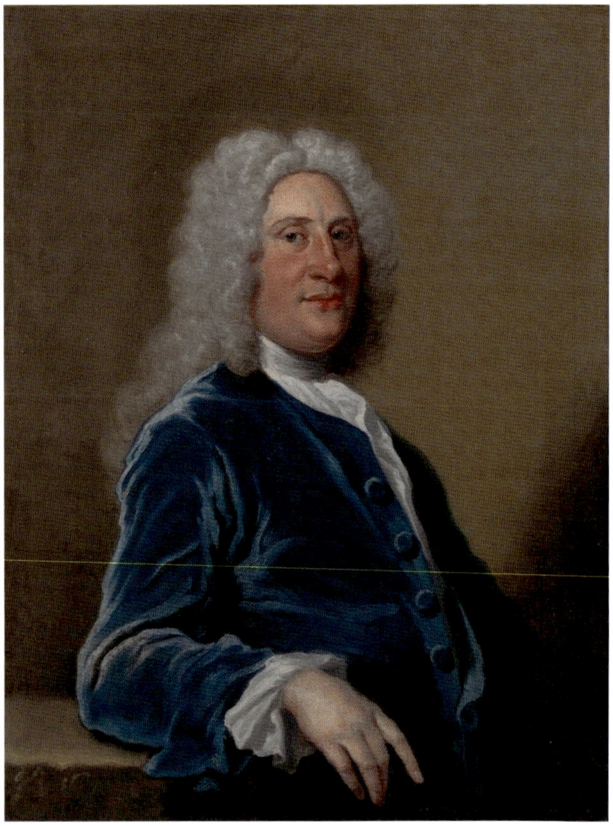

13 Joseph Highmore, *Unknown Man*, between 1730 and 1735, oil on canvas, 91.4 x 71.1 cm, Yale Centre for British Art, Paul Mellon Collection

Significantly, through his membership, Highmore was also introduced to important freemasons who were prominent participants in the creation of a new chivalric order, the Order of the Bath. In the *Memoirs*, having mentioned Highmore's move to Lincoln's Inn Fields, John Duncombe notes that 'an opportunity soon offered of introducing him advantageously to the nobility, &c. by his being desired, by Mr. Pine the engraver, to make the drawings for his prints of the Knights of the Bath, on the revival of that order, in 1725'.[54] Aside from Sir Robert Walpole, the first 'prime minister' and a freemason, the most noteworthy member, after royalty, was the first Great Master of the order John Montagu, 2nd Duke of Montagu (Great Master 1725–49), who had been the Grand Master of the freemasons from 1721 to 1723. Similarly Charles Lennox, 2nd Duke of Richmond and William O'Brian, Earl of Inchiquin, both created Knight Companions of the Order of the Bath in 1725, were Grand Master of the freemasons in 1724 and 1726 respectively. At the very least, the masonic connections gave Highmore a competitive edge over non-mason artists.

That the Bath project assisted in achieving Highmore's aim of gaining access to the social elite more generally is evident from the noticeable increase in aristocratic portraits produced by Highmore from the late 1720s (fig. 13).[55] However, according to the *Memoirs*, an event of even greater significance had occurred as part of, or deriving from, the Order of the Bath. After introducing Pine's project as one that had provided the artist with an opportunity to introduce himself to the nobility – that is, 'in consequence, several of the knights had their portraits also by the same hand' – the paragraph concludes: 'And our artist was sent for to St. James's, by King George I. to draw the late Duke of Cumberland, from which Smith scraped a mezzotinto'.[56]

'HIS FAVOURITE MASTER'

Having broadened his client base to include aristocracy and even royalty, the most important events in the early 1730s were Highmore's two foreign journeys. The first, in 1732, to the Low Countries and Düsseldorf, was probably his first trip to continental Europe. The second, in 1734, was to Paris.[57] Although the royal and aristocratic collections located in London, its environs and in scores of country estates throughout Britain were available for artists to study, the depth and breadth of experience acquired through travel abroad was deemed vital to their education and refinement. As an artist who valued every opportunity to expand his contacts, as well as his knowledge and experience, it is unsurprising that Highmore took full advantage when his professional circumstances permitted.

The *Memoirs* state that

> In the summer of 1732, Mr. Highmore visited the continent, in company with Dr. Pemberton, Mr. Benj. Robins, and two other friends, chiefly with a view to

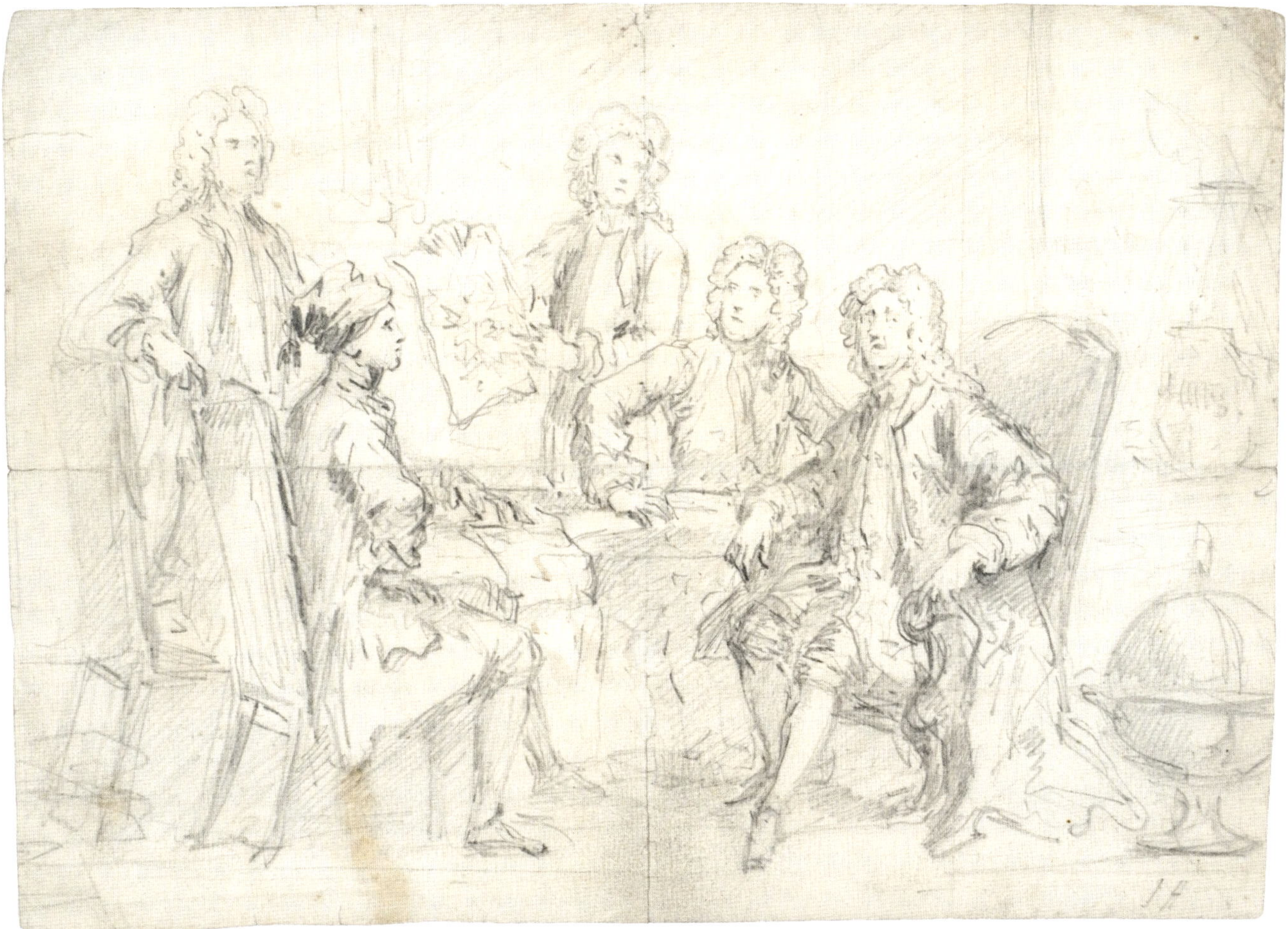

14 Joseph Highmore, *Sketch of a group of five gentlemen around a table*, date not known, graphite on paper, 207 x 293 mm, Tate

The five men surround a table covered in maps, with a globe (bottom right) and ship (top right). The central standing figure is holding up a ground plan of a fortification, which may identify him as the ballistics expert Benjamin Robins. This could therefore be a sketch for a formal, commemorative group portrait of the friends' 1732 trip to the Low Countries, with Robins, Henry Pemberton, their two unnamed companions and Highmore, the latter seated to the left wearing a cap.

seeing the gallery of the pictures belonging to the Elector Palatine at Dusseldorp, collected by Rubens, and supposed the best in Europe. At Antwerp also he had peculiar pleasure in contemplating the works of his favourite master. In their return they visited the principal towns in Holland.[58]

This brief passage is all that is currently known of the purpose and itinerary of the journey. Highmore's two identified companions were Henry Pemberton (1694–1771), a mathematician, associate of Sir Isaac Newton and fellow of the Royal Society, and Benjamin Robins (1707–1751), a mathematician specializing in fortifications and ballistics and like Pemberton a member of the Royal Society (fig. 14).[59]

Returning to the *Memoirs*, the 'principal towns in Holland' must have included Amsterdam, the city most associated with Rembrandt van Rijn (1606–1669). Highmore had a strong interest in Rembrandt. His sale catalogue includes 'A Lady Abbess, in the Manner of *Rembrandt*' and 'A large Head, after *Rembrandt*', both by Highmore himself.[60] Neither painting is traced, but it can be assumed that both displayed a close study of Rembrandt's technique and composition, as the following observation by Highmore indicates: 'Those who are acquainted with the works of Rembrandt, will see ... his tints are so pure, so little mixed or compounded, and his pictures so remarkably strong and clear, and never change or decay'.[61] The other Dutch cities can be guessed at. In preparation for *An Account of some of the Statues, Bas-reliefs, Drawing and Pictures in Italy, &c* (published 1722) Jonathan Richardson the Younger travelled to Rotterdam, Leiden, The Hague and Brussels, and, while stressing in his notes examples of Italian art, observed that a majority of the paintings in these collections were by Dutch and Flemish artists.[62]

The fact that Rubens is mentioned twice within the short account in the *Memoirs* is significant. Highmore's high opinion of Rubens – something of a passion – is confirmed by the phrase 'his favourite master'. Further, the description of Highmore as 'contemplating' Rubens's works in Antwerp rather than 'viewing' them suggests a lingering focus on his part. Such experience, dependent on particular and exclusive access to major examples of Rubens's work unequalled in London or Britain (the ceiling of the Banqueting House, Whitehall aside) allowed Highmore to develop, in turn, a particular knowledge of the great Flemish artist's *oeuvre* and technique. Highmore's admiration extended to the collecting and painting of works after Rubens. His sale catalogue includes '*The* Graces *unveiling* Nature, after Rubens', '*Rubens*'s Wife, from an Original at *Antwerp*', both by Highmore. It also contains 'A Bacchanalian of Boys in a Landscape' and 'The Venus Genitrix', both listed as after Rubens but not attributed in this source to Highmore.[63] As with the works he had executed in the style of or after Rembrandt, the existence of these paintings in Highmore's studio confirms his close study of Rubens's compositions and technique.

The two cities named in the *Memoirs*, Düsseldorf and Antwerp, were also visited and recorded by Richardson the Younger. Antwerp was Rubens's home and where he built his palatial residence and studio.[64] However, no specific location, collection or painting in the city is named in the *Memoirs*. It should be noted that Antwerp was also associated with Sir Anthony van Dyck, Jacob Jordaens (1593–1678), Jan Brueghel the Elder (1568–1625) and Younger (1601–1678) and David Teniers I (1582–1649) and II (1610–1690). Yet Rubens alone is named in the *Memoirs* in relation to Antwerp, confirming Highmore's partiality for him.

In regard to the Elector Palatine's Gallery at Düsseldorf, Richardson comments, 'Rubens is Here seen in Perfection: I believe there is about 40 Pictures of him, many very Capital', and, later, 'Whoever sees this Collection must have a Greater Idea of Rubens that 'tis possible to have without seeing it; and such a One as will give him a place amongst the most Excellent Painters'.[65] A near contemporary catalogue of the art displayed in the Elector Palatine's Gallery, written by Gerard Joseph Karsch and published c.1725, offers a comprehensive guide to the works that Highmore would have seen in 1732. Among the Rubens paintings that Richardson had praised so highly were *The Fall of the Damned* (1620–21), *The Great Last Judgment* (1617), *The Battle of the Amazons* (1617–18), *The Death of Seneca* (1612/13) and, in portraiture, the artist's *Self-portrait with Isabella Brandt ('The Honeysuckle Bower'*; 1609–10), all now in the Alte Pinakothek, Munich.[66]

Highmore was to return to the Continent only two years later and the resulting journal, with its quick notes, sketches and observations, remains, as earlier stated, the single most important document written by him. Highmore spent two and half months away from London, departing by packet from the Tower on Sunday 2 June 1734 and returning on Tuesday 13 August.[67] A majority of this time was spent in Paris itself and its immediate environs. Highmore's unguarded response to the art he saw, as recounted in this unedited and private format, is particularly revealing. In some cases his negative, almost dismissive response to works by Italian artists, considered by many of his peers – most notably Richardson Senior and Junior – as the prime models for emulation, offers proof of an independence of thought, perhaps even a subversive streak. This, coupled with the prominence of Flemish art, specifically Rubens, in his choice of itinerary and corresponding notations suggests that the Paris trip acted as an adjunct to his earlier experience in the Low Countries and Düsseldorf.

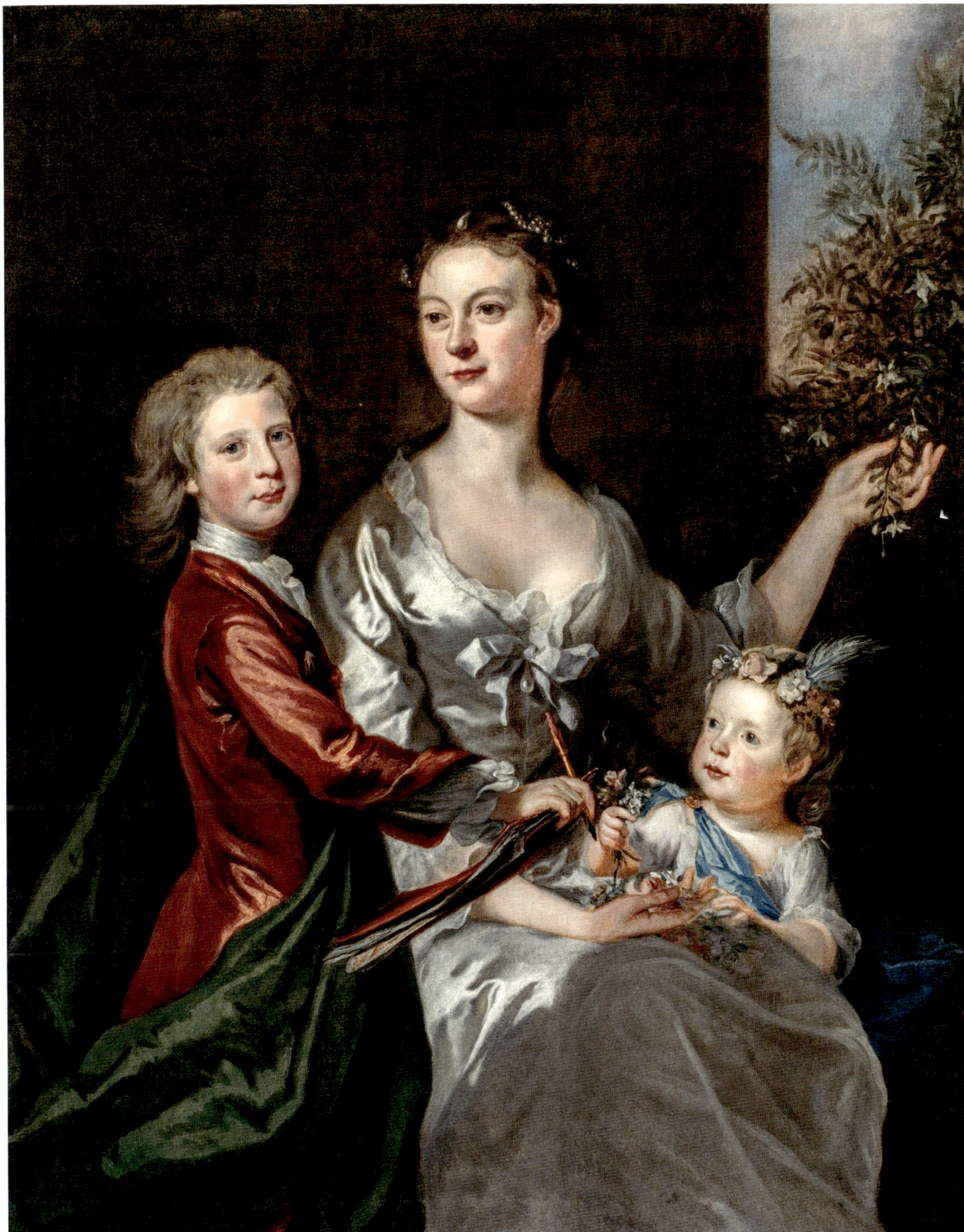

15 Joseph Highmore, *The Artist's Wife Susanna, Son Anthony and Daughter Susanna*, London, c.1728, oil on canvas, 126 x 101.7 cm, Art Gallery of South Australia, Adelaide, Gift of the Art Gallery of South Australia Foundation, 1994

Highmore's itinerary also demonstrates an interest in meeting prominent members of the Académie Royale de peinture et sculpture and in viewing examples of recent and contemporary French art.

Offering just an indication of the breadth, variety and at times exclusivity of Highmore's art-related visits, his schedule included the royal palaces of the Louvre, Luxembourg (twice), Bourbon, Palais-Royal (twice), Versailles and Marly; the Hôtels Lambert, Bouillon, d'Antin, Richelieu; the Hôtel de Ville, the Sorbonne, the Hôtel des Invalides, the Gobelins Tapestry factory and the Royal Observatory; the churches of Notre Dame, St-Sulpice, St-Roch, St- Symphorien and the Carmelites and the convent of the Capucines; the Académie Royale (located in the Louvre; twice); the studios of the sculptor and draughtsman Edmé Bouchardon (1698–1762), the still-life painter and tapestry designer Jean-Baptiste Oudry (1686–1755), the history painter Jean II Restout (1692–1768), the *fêtes galantes* painter Nicolas Lancret (1690–1743), the history painter Nöel-Nicolas Coypel (1690–1734), his nephew, *le premier peintre du roi* Charles-Antoine Coypel (1694–1752), the portrait painters Hyacinthe Rigaud (1659–1743), Nicolas de Largillière (1656–1746) and Carle van Loo (1705–1765); and several private collections including those of Pierre Dubreuil, jeweller, *écuyer et premier valet de chambre de la reine* (twice); Pierre Crozat (1661–1740), the financier, art collector and patron of Jean-Antoine Watteau (three times); Cardinal Melchior de Polignac (1661–1741), former ambassador to Rome; and the duc de Tallard, governor of Franche-Comté. Most of these visits were completed in the first three weeks that Highmore was in Paris.

According to brief notes at the back of the journal, Highmore carried letters of recommendation, private correspondence and business-related letters from at least five associates in London, including Peter Daudé, nephew of the Huguenot mathematician Pierre Daudé (1653–1733).[68] The first art-related letter was from the Paris-born engraver and draughtsman Hubert François Bourguignon, known as Gravelot (1699–1773), to his sister. Highmore dined with Gravelot's family and made several visits to important collections in the company of his father and brother.[69] The second art-related letter was from the sculptor Louis-François Roubiliac to the Académie Royale professor and *sculpteur du roi* Jacques Bousseau (1681–1740). Like Gravelot, Roubiliac had recently arrived in London. Bousseau probably acted as Highmore's sponsor and guide on his two visits to the Académie Royale.[70]

Highmore visited Versailles over a three-day period in the lively company of Dr Nathaniel Hickman, the tutor of the Duke of Kingston and a well-known art connoisseur or *amateur*. There they observed King Louis XV 'at Mass & after at Din[ne]r' and later returning from hunting. Another entry declares that his companions 'told King of me'.[71] After viewing Charles de la Fosse's *Moses saved from the Waters* (dated between 1675 and 1680), Highmore declared La Fosse (1636–1716) to be 'ye best of all ye French mas[te]rs for Colrg drapery Composition tout ensemble'.[72] The following day Highmore noted: 'This morning at ye Kings Levee, went with him to Mass again, saw there the Dauphine. whom I saw brought back in a chair thro the apartem[en]ts a fine sprightly jolly countenance'. Highmore then viewed 'the great Oval of Mr Le Moine', that is *The Apotheosis of Hercules* of 1733–36. Highmore conversed with François Lemoyne (1688–1737) on two occasions while Lemoyne was painting 'on his Scaffold' in the Salon d'Hercule, noting 'I think him the ablest painter I have seen in all respects'.[73]

On his return to Paris, Highmore visited the Palais du Luxembourg for the second time. In his *Dialogue on Colouring*, the French artist and theorist Roger de Piles (1635–1709) stated: 'the best Counsel I can give a Painter (if I were capable of giving him any) shou'd be once a Week for a space of a Year to visit the Gallery of Luxembourg, to lay all things else aside, and to spare nothing for that purpose. That day wou'd be undoubtedly the best spent of any in the Week.'[74] The gallery mentioned contained the Marie des Médicis canvases by Rubens (painted c.1621–25). Highmore clearly took de Piles's advice to heart. In fact he was so keen to see the Rubens paintings that he had visited the palace on his first full day in Paris. From his journal we know that Highmore was familiar with the twenty-four engravings after these works which had been published by Bernard Picart and others as a complete volume in 1710, and he appears to have made a particular study of them before leaving London for Paris. On his first visit Highmore notes:

> the Pictures very different some excellent in ye highest degree particularly l'accouchemt de la Reine tho' her face seems somewhat damaged, the figure who holds the child in ye greatest perfection of colouring & drawing. That representing ye City of Lyons undoubtedly of his own hand the Boy on ye further lyon the finest I ever saw [small sketch by Highmore here] This & ye former I think ye 2 best.[75]

Highmore was less impressed by *The Council of the Gods*: 'That where Apollo is towards at the Bottom of the picture (& ye other Deities being above) not equal to my Expectation this with several others seem not all of his own Execution'.[76] These observations reveal Highmore's confidence in being able to separate Rubens's hand from those of his students or later restorers. Given the time and attention he had spent scrutinizing 'his favourite master', including venturing to see the magnificent Rubens collection in Düsseldorf, he had every reason to be confident.

As a portrait-painter, Highmore seems to have particularly relished visiting the studios of the esteemed academicians Hyacinthe Rigaud and Nicolas de Largillière, who were both Académie Royale contemporaries of the Great Queen Street directors Louis Chéron and Louis Laguerre (1663–1721). They were known primarily for portraiture, yet both had branched out successfully into history painting, as Highmore, in one of the longest entries in his journal, observes with evident interest:

> Largiliere ... has been an excellent painter of Portraits besides w[hi]ch has discovered an extraordinary Genius for History of wch many in his House all painted without the life well composed particularly with regard to the lights and shadow in wch he has succeeded marvellously and in various manners. Rigaud has also painted of History but very few, more correct than the other but less fire & freedom too much of the lay man.[77]

Without doubt, Highmore's Continental experiences during the 1730s and the stimulation he gained through visiting the Académie Royale and engaging with his French peers would have provided an impetus to vary his practice to include other genres, specifically history painting. It would also have spurred him to introduce greater variety and invention, where possible, into his portraiture. In fact, not long after his return from Paris, Highmore had the opportunity to do both.

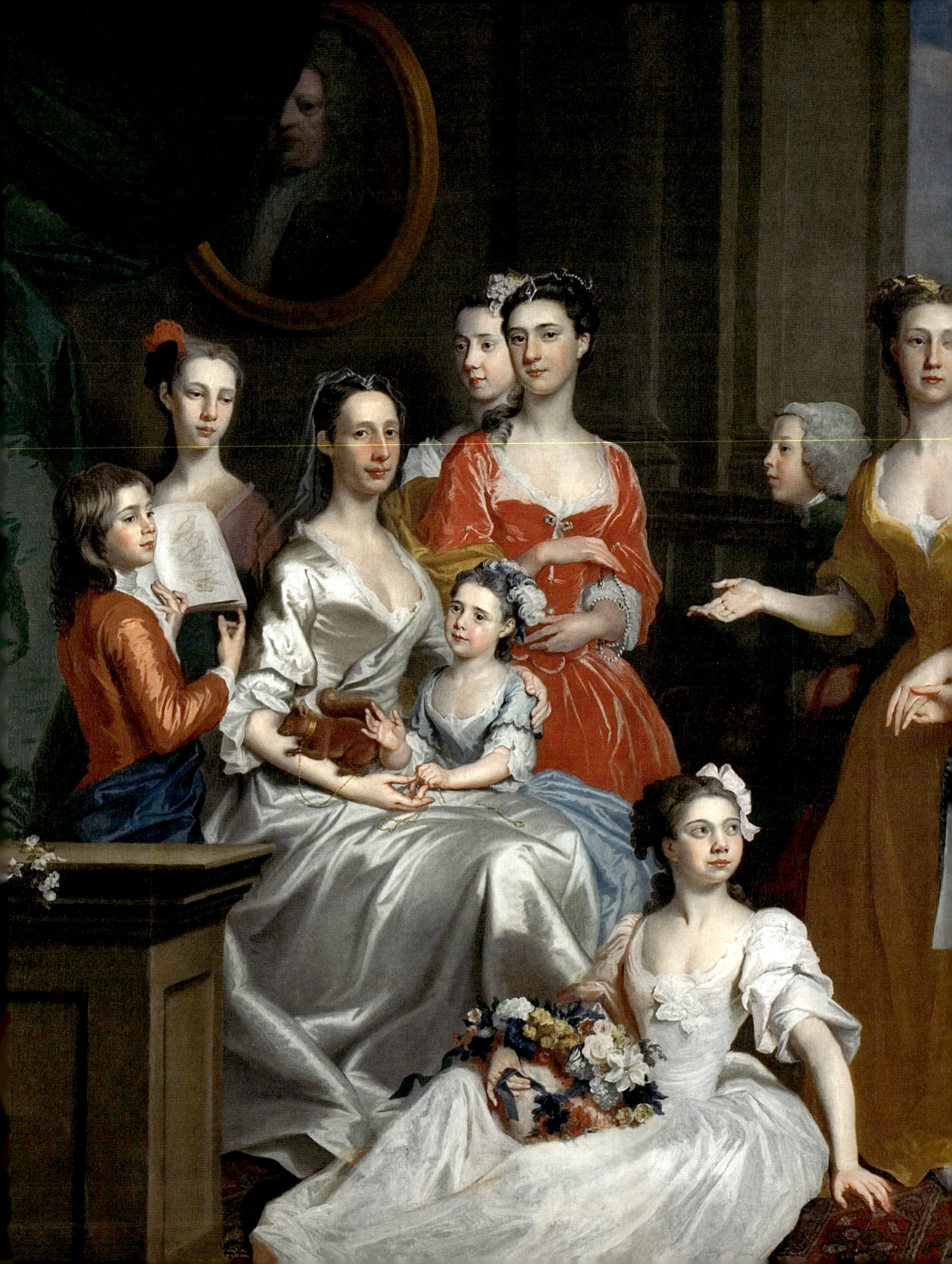

'THE CONFIDENCE OF FRIENDSHIP AND THE TENDERNESS OF LOVE'

In his summary of the first ten years of Highmore's career, George Vertue had noted that the artist had 'good employ' among the citizens of the City of London, going on to observe that 'he had made many family pieces. heads. &c.'.[1] Over sixty years later, Highmore's son-in-law, the Rev. John Duncombe, wrote: 'his knowledge of perspective gave him great advantages in family-pieces, of which he painted more than any one of his time'.[2] Both authors draw attention to family portraiture as a core strand within Highmore's practice, while Vertue's separation of 'family pieces' from 'heads. &c.' makes a distinction between portraits of individual members – standard format, single sitter, the mainstay of any portrait practice – and the family within groups or as a whole, that is, 'family pieces'. Combinations of husband and wife, of mother and child or children, or of siblings, and in standard portrait formats, are certainly not unusual within Highmore's oeuvre.

Yet Duncombe's comment concerning perspective would have little bearing on them. This reference, used specifically in regard to the term 'family pieces', can only apply to a format that required the skilful placing of a series of individuals at full-length and within an interior or exterior space, a format typified by the small-scale canvases now loosely termed 'conversation pieces'.[3] If the family pieces, as described by Vertue, were indeed 'conversations', then this might reflect the modest ambition of Highmore's early City-based clients – merchants, schoolmasters, clergymen, civic leaders – relative to the traditional large-scale aristocratic group portraiture of Sir Anthony Van Dyck and Sir Godfrey Kneller. It would also establish Highmore's early usage of this newly imported, informal portrait style.[4] That, by the time he retired, Highmore had painted more of these portraits than any artist of his generation is quite a claim, given the competition for such an accolade from, among others, William Hogarth and Philippe Mercier (1689–1760).

In any case, considering Vertue and Duncombe's observations, it would be a fair assumption that multi-figure family portraits would form a significant portion of Highmore's output. However, only one life-sized full-length group, *The Family of Sir Eldred Lancelot Lee* (1736; see fig. 25), and three small-scale conversations are currently known – the painting of Highmore's own family (see fig. 6); *The Vigor Family* of 1744 (see fig. 33); and *The Whichcote Wedding* of 1749 (current location unknown, but still with the Whichcote family in 1963).[5] The small painting known as *'John Rich and Family'* (fig. 21), which is dateable to the late 1720s or early 1730s, is probably an oil sketch for a larger portrait. Similarly, the painting at the Yale Center for British Art (fig. 16) appears to be a preparatory oil sketch, produced to set out the figures of an extended family group within a formal garden-terrace setting. Whether for a final composition on a small or large scale, Highmore's use of perspective is demonstrated within the architectural elements, including the flooring, and in the overall sense of depth.

However, with the two client-commissioned conversations dated to the mid and late 1740s, this means that no 'family piece' from Highmore's early career (pre-1725) is currently known. Yet the many sketches of family groups in the Highmore Family Gift (figs. 2, 3, 5, 10, 11, 14, 17, 18 and 82) seem to support Vertue and Duncombe's claim that this portrait type

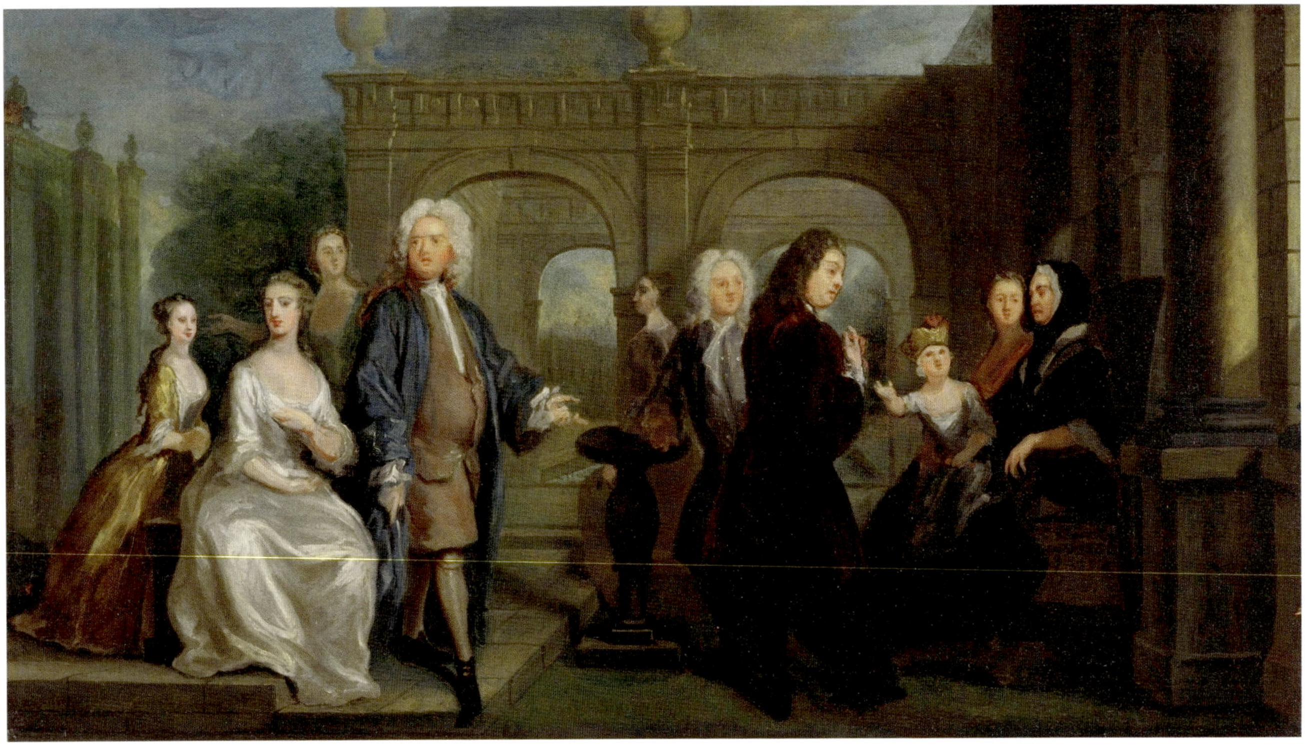

16 Joseph Highmore, *A Family Conversation Piece*, between 1730 and 1735, oil on canvas, 45.1 x 80 cm, Yale Center for British Art, Paul Mellon Collection

was a significant one throughout his career. Given the unknown recent history of *The Whichcote Wedding* and the 'discovery' of the Vigor portrait – unrecorded until it was acquired by the Victoria and Albert Museum in 2009 – one explanation is that such paintings, small in scale and easily accommodated within modern interiors, remain with descendants of the family who commissioned them and have not yet emerged into public notice, for example via the saleroom. The five paintings and oil sketches named above are important examples of a potentially significant but currently little known element of Highmore's practice.

This chapter will therefore focus on a series of case studies, with an emphasis on three types of family portraiture produced by Highmore: the first is the 'group' portrait formed by the creation and assembly of individual or double portraits; the second is the large group portrait on a single canvas; and the third the conversation or family piece. Regarding the first, the portraits commissioned by Robert Warner (c.1705–1765) and James Harris (1709–1780) offer a rare insight into Highmore's adoption by socially connected families that fall, in this instance, within the professional and propertied 'middling sort'. The relationship can be traced through an exchange of letters between Harris, his friend Warner and Highmore himself, some held in the Malmesbury Family Archive (Hampshire Record Office).[6] A majority of the extracts are published here for the first time. The correspondence reveals practical details relating to Highmore's portraiture, such as his system of pricing, as well as the day-to-day dynamics between painter and patron, patron and portrait. Meanwhile, *The Lee Family* presents both an intricate visual record of two generations of this family from the Shropshire landed gentry and an ambitious representation of ancestry and dynasty. Finally, the focus will move from the monumental to the small-scale intimacy of *The Vigor Family*. Collectively,

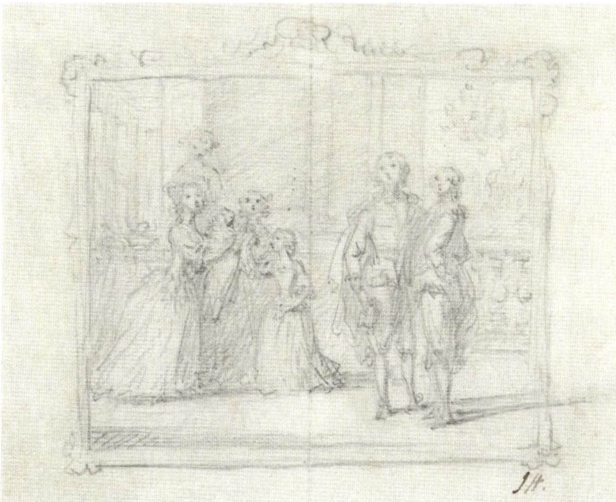

17 Joseph Highmore, *A family group of seven persons standing on a terrace*, date not known, graphite on paper, 152 x 184 mm, Tate

The male figures to the right are dressed and posed in the seventeenth-century 'Van Dyck' manner, a portrait style Highmore used throughout the 1730s and 1740s (see fig. 19). No oil on canvas connected to this sketch is currently known.

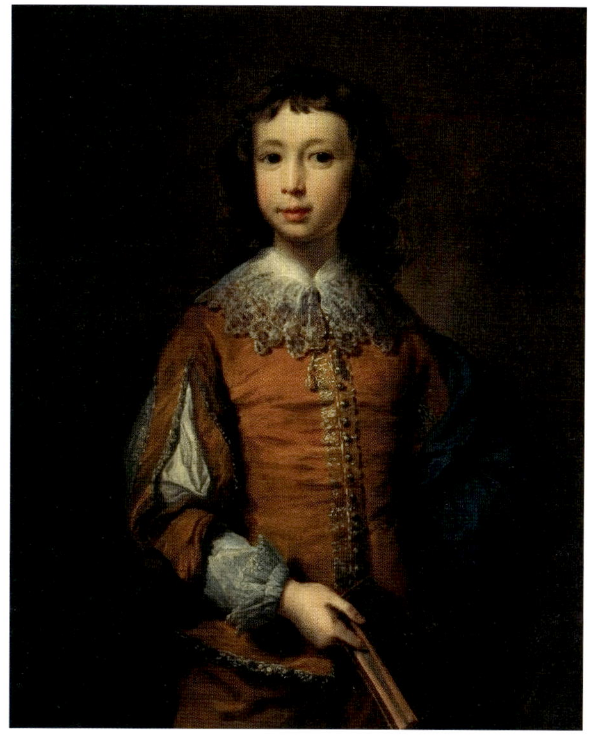

19 Joseph Highmore, *A Boy in Van Dyck Costume*, 1748, oil on canvas, 73 x 60.5 cm, Waddesdon Manor, Buckinghamshire

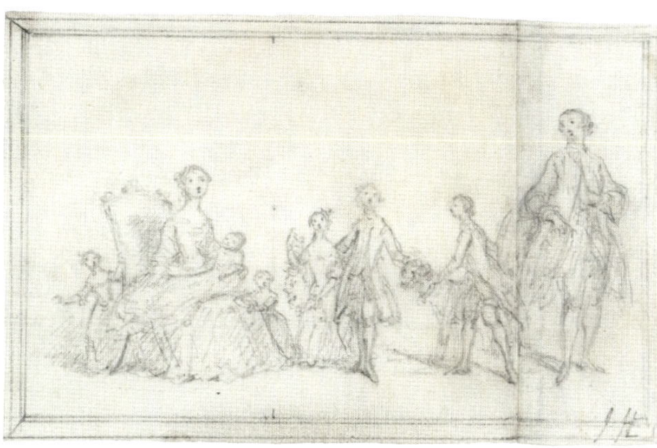

18 Joseph Highmore, *A family group of eight persons and a dog, full-length*, date not known, graphite on paper, 108 x 169 mm, Tate

and in tandem with issues of status and individual circumstance, the examples explored here shed light on bonds of friendship, love and esteem within social and family groups, as expressed through the versatile medium of portraiture.

'DELIVER'D DOWN TO POSTERITY'

By the 1730s Robert Warner and James Harris lived mainly in Hampshire, the former at Anstey near Alton and the latter in Salisbury, although they had professional and family connections in London. According to John Nichols, in his *Literary Anecdotes of the Eighteenth Century*, Robert's brother Richard (1713?–1775), a botanist and literary scholar, was originally 'bred to the law, and for some time had chambers in Lincoln's Inn'.[7] In fact, Robert, James Harris and the latter's brother Thomas had all been members of Lincoln's Inn, revealing that Highmore's early career in law

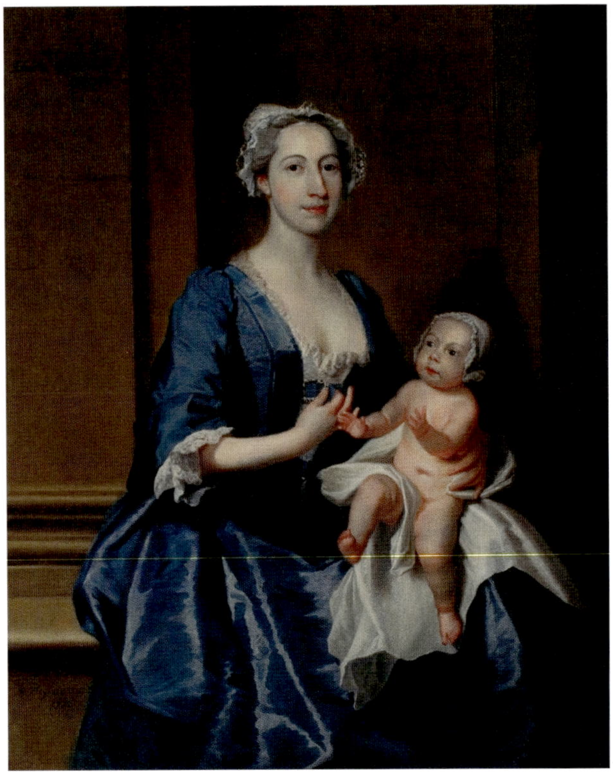

20 Joseph Highmore, *Johanna Warner and her Son John*, 1736, oil on canvas, 127 x 101.6 cm, on loan to Mottisfont Abbey, Hampshire

continued to be a source for portrait commissions long after he abandoned it.[8] Highmore's studio, close to the chambers of Lincoln's Inn, was certainly convenient for sittings and the exchange of letters. However, as Highmore was one of several artists living in the area, it is likely that this group turned to him because they admired his portrait style, finding it wholly compatible with their needs and self-image, as well as through friendship and a sense of loyalty.

In July 1737, Robert Warner wrote to James Harris that 'Highmore hath taken mine my wife's & her sons Picture & Mr. Leighs, you shall see them at his House'.[9] The whereabouts of Robert Warner's portrait is currently unknown, but the painting of his wife Johanna née Leigh and infant son, John Leigh Warner (b. 1736), passed into the collection of Robert's descendants, the Clarke-Jervoise family, and is now at Mottisfont Abbey, Hampshire (fig. 20). Johanna is shown serenely balancing her chubby, wriggling infant on her knee. The abstract shimmer of her mid-blue silk robe contrasts with the severe stone architecture, which in turn draws attention to the pink flesh-tints of the naked child and the paler tones of Johanna's face, décolletage and raised right arm. There is the hint of a smile on Johanna's face, which seems to combine the pride and anxiety of a new mother. The visually dominant use of blue and white for Johanna's clothing and the fabric that partially covers her son might reflect the traditional 'colour coding' of the Madonna and Child. It is repeated in '*John Rich and Family*' (fig. 21). That this is a realistic rather than overly flattering portrayal is suggested by Johanna's naturally grey hair.

Although its current location is also unknown, the third portrait mentioned by Robert, that of his brother-in-law Barnabas Eveleigh Leigh (b. 1703), remained with the same Warner descendants until 1977.[10] From a black-and-white sale catalogue photograph we know that Barnabas stands against a plain, dark background, which, unlike Johanna's portrait, has been given an extra element of luxury through the inclusion of a silk drape. According to the lot description, Barnabas's velvet coat is red.[11] He turns his body towards the left, with his right hand gesturing in the same direction, perhaps (if the intention, from the onset, was to hang the portraits together) towards his sister, while lightly placing his left hand on a volume of the works of the classical Roman poet Horace that rests on a stone plinth beside him. The prominence of the book draws attention to the sitter's literary and intellectual interests. The portraits of Johanna Warner and her brother Barnabas Leigh are both 'half-lengths' (50 × 40 inches) and signed and dated 1736. It is likely therefore that Robert's portrait was of the same size and format. As John is shown as a baby in the double portrait, it was surely the birth of Robert and Johanna's first child, Robert's son and heir, which prompted the formation of a family picture gallery.

Later, in 1738, Robert Warner writes, again to James Harris:

> I very narrowly missed ye Pleasure of our Friend Highmore's company here for a day or two, he was set out

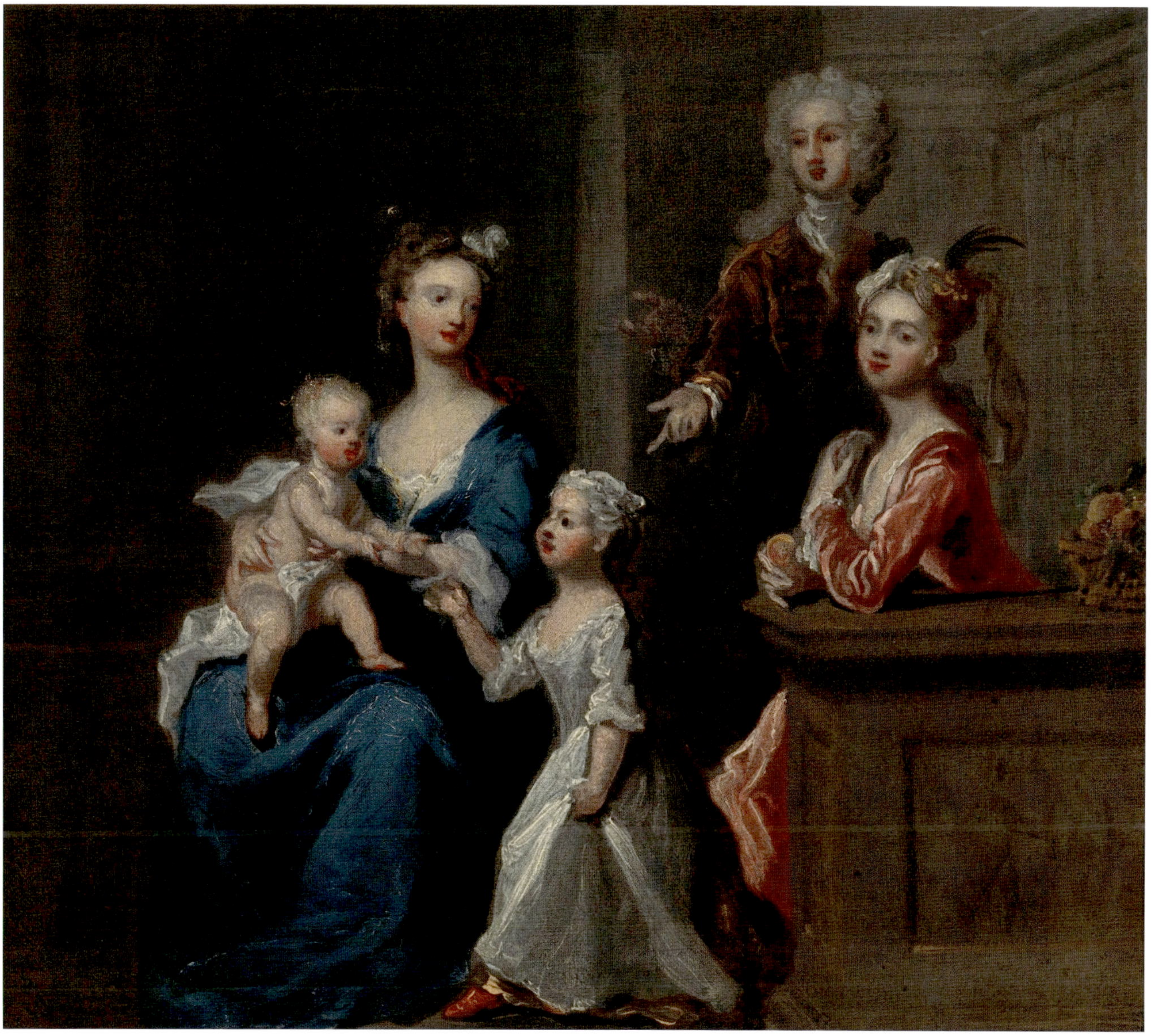

21 Joseph Highmore, Group portrait called *'John Rich and Family'*, late 1720s/early 1730s, oil on canvas, 29.2 x 33 cm, The Garrick Club, London

> but an accident happened to his horse which prevented him, he has made my Parlour very Agreeable by four Family Pictures, one of which my Brother Richards is I think well worth your seeing.[12]

Note Robert's use of the term 'family picture' for a standard portrait of a family member. Robert also informs James Harris that all four paintings of the Warner-Leigh family – the husband, wife and son, brother-in-law and now the brother – were hanging together in the same room, no doubt as planned, creating an immediate and visually impressive family gallery, representing the current generation and the beginnings of the next.

Richard's portrait is also untraced, but some sense of its appearance and effect is suggested by Robert's comment to James Harris that it is 'well worth your seeing'. In a letter written by John Hoadly (1711–1776), son of Bishop Benjamin Hoadly, to Richard, dated 26 April 1744, John jests: 'have You too great a Respect for ye French, our natural Enemies? I myself have seen You in a French Wastcoat; nay, more, such was your Love for it, that you are deliver'd down to Posterity, by ye. Hand of ye great Highmore, in that Habiliment.'[13] John's reference to 'our natural Enemies' may be an allusion to the failed French invasion, earlier that year, to restore the exiled Catholic Stuarts to the throne of Great Britain. Even so, Richard's French waistcoat was clearly remarkable for its Continental flamboyance. As a result, John teasingly accuses his friend of presenting himself to the world, and indeed posterity, as a bit of a dandy. There is also a suggestion – just a hint – that for this social group there was a nagging feeling that the commissioning of a portrait might smack of vanity.

'THE APPROBATION OF YOUR FRIENDS'

In a letter dated 4 June 1738 Robert Warner wrote to James Harris that 'Highmore is going to revisit Antwerp, if I was not marryed[,] if I were not marryed much to my liking[,] I would go with him. A Single Life has that Advantage one may much easyer Dispatriate.'[14] As far as is known, Highmore did not return to Antwerp, but this comment hints at the possibility that Robert Warner was one of the two unnamed men who joined Highmore in his 1732 trip to the Low Countries.

In the same year as Robert's letter, Highmore was commissioned to paint the portrait of James Harris's long-deceased grandfather. The production of such 'ancestral' portraiture was unusual within Highmore's practice. Harris's maternal grandfather was Anthony Ashley Cooper, 2nd Earl of Shaftesbury (1652–1699), and James was therefore nephew to the 3rd Earl, the celebrated author of the theoretical text *Characteristicks* (1711).[15] However, it can now be confirmed that the portrait commissioned was of Harris's paternal grandfather Thomas Harris (1643–1679). The Malmesbury collection also includes a bust-length portrait of Thomas Harris's second wife, Joan née Wyndham (m. 1673, d. 1734; daughter of Sir Wadham Wyndham of Orchard Wyndham), attributed to Mary Beale. By family tradition the two portraits hang together, despite the male sitter being misidentified as Joan's son (James Harris's father, also James) rather than her husband. The similarity in format and the posing of the two sitters, facing towards each other, suggest that Harris commissioned Highmore to produce an image that acted as a pendant to his grandmother's much earlier portrait. Her recent death, aged eighty-four, may have been the stimulus.[16]

That James Harris, with the commissioning of his grandfather's portrait, was contemplating the formation of a family gallery is borne out by Harris's subsequent commissions. In early July 1740 Highmore refers to a portrait of James Harris himself, which the painter tells him is completed, but awaiting its frame and packing case for transportation to Salisbury.[17] This portrait (fig. 22) also remains in the Malmesbury collection. Harris is portrayed in a mid-length white wig and a mid-grey velvet housecoat with a plain, white shirt and stock. He looks out to his right, his right hand elegantly raised, while leaning with his left on a plain brown stone plinth. No attribute, such as a book, is included, despite Harris's now leisured existence and literary ambitions.[18] The background is plain, allowing the strong light that enters from the

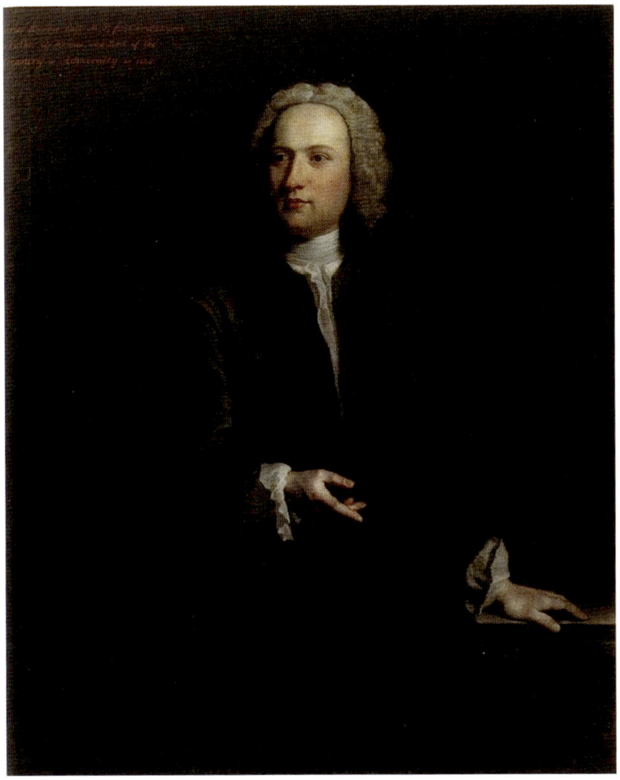

22 Joseph Highmore, *James Harris*, 1740, oil on canvas, 127 x 101.6 cm, Malmesbury Collection

top right to highlight the face, body and plinth. The palette, limited to white, grey and brown, together with the lighting, draws the eye to the face and James's character. On 30 July 1740 Highmore wrote, from Lincoln's Inn Fields, 'I am very glad that your Portrait <has> met with the approbation of your friends that have seen it here, and shall be proud to understand that those at Salisbury differ not from them'.[19] Certainly, from a business point of view, the display of the portrait in London and then Salisbury expanded the potential for new clients among Harris's friends and associates immeasurably.

Two years later James Harris commissioned a portrait of his father, James Harris (1674–1731). James Harris Junior inherited the family estate on his father's death, including the main residence, designed by Sir Christopher Wren, at St Anne's Gate, the Close, Salisbury (now Malmesbury House). At the end of March 1742 Highmore wrote that the portrait of Harris's father 'is now totally finish'd unless you will give me leave to shew a little gold where the waistcoat discover's it's self under the coat? also wo.d <you> have any thing on the table, w.ch I have cover'd with crimson?'[20] Highmore's proposal to add some luxury to the portrait, through the hint of a gold waistcoat, suggests that, aesthetically, it might lift an otherwise unfussy costume. Even so, the degree of restraint or extravagance, as we have seen with Richard Warner's portrait, would be the client's choice. Again, the query 'wo.d <you> have any thing on the table ... ?' reveals a professional leading a client through the options available, in this instance the inclusion of an object or attribute that will add a biographical layer and visual interest. Highmore's pricing for this 'half-length' is ten guineas 'as every thing is new but the face',[21] confirming that Highmore was basing his portrait on an existing image.

By 1742, and through his own efforts, James Harris's private collection at St Anne's Gate now contained images of himself, his father and paternal grandfather, all by the same artist. However, and in imitation of Robert Warner's commissions in 1736, after James's marriage in 1745 Highmore painted a half-length of his bride Elizabeth and three years later a double portrait of Elizabeth and her young son, James's heir, both of which remain with the family. Although the correspondence between Harris and Highmore continued well into the 1760s, as far as is known James did not commission any further family portraits from him. Those of Harris's other surviving children Gertrude (b. 1750) and Louisa (b. 1753) are by George Romney and dated 1777. Even so, Harris's patronage of Highmore, apparently to the exclusion of any other portrait painter during that time, spanned ten years.

Highmore's portrait of James Harris did indeed generate interest among his friends when it arrived in Salisbury, as the painter had hoped. In 1741 Highmore responded to a query by Henry Wyndham, resident at the College, Salisbury, and distantly related to James Harris (through Harris's grandmother), regarding prices:

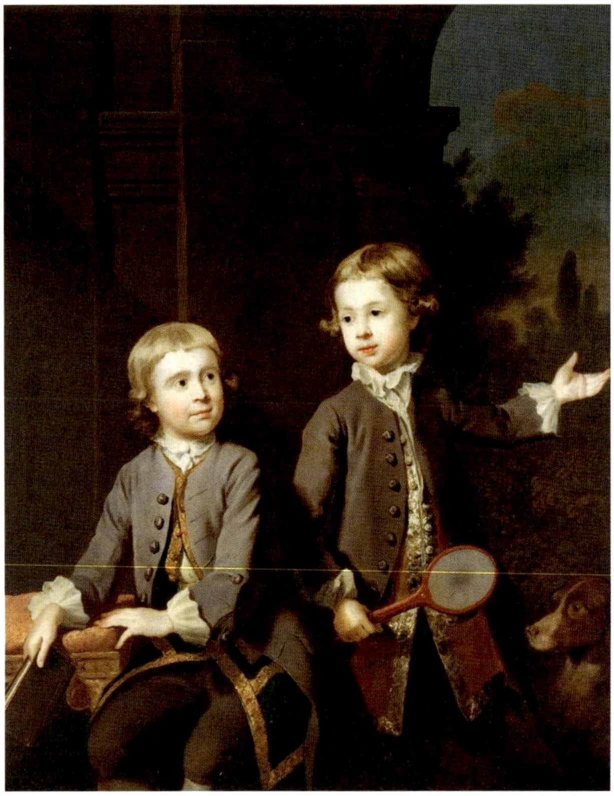

23 Joseph Highmore, *Double Portrait of Henry Penruddocke Wyndham and his Brother Wadham*, 1743, oil on canvas, 127 x 101.5 cm, private collection

Henry later became Mayor of Salisbury and Whig MP for Wiltshire, while Wadham joined the British Army and acquired some fame as a *bon vivant*. The contrast in temperament is already clear in Highmore's portrait.

> In answer to your question from Mr. Wyndham – the price of a copy is always half that of an original – if it were the size of your Portrait (as the original wo.[d] be 20 Guineas) the copy wo.[d] be 10. thô I have generally 15. when the copy is taken from a smaller, because then all the Posture &c: is original, however I don't insist on that.[22]

Highmore goes on to confirm his pricing for single portraits: 'I have not painted under the rates of 10. 20. and 40 G.[s] [guineas] for heads, half lengths, and whole = lengths these eighteen years'. As Wyndham's query also concerns Highmore's charge for a portrait that contains more than one figure, but is the same size as a 'single' portrait, he continues with a lengthy explanation of his method and prices. The passage provides invaluable information as to how a painter of this period balanced the cost of labour and materials with issues of design and effect:

> in family pictures the composition may vary the price by the disposition of parts, because the way of computing is by whole length, half, and head, – Where only two persons are to make a picture (besides that the architecture &c: will be as much or more than if a greater number where [sic] in the same picture), it wo.[d] not be so agreable that one sho.[d] hide half of the other without any apparent reason, such disposition however wo.[d] reduce the price from 80. to 60. G.[s] according to the rule laid down: the last of this kind I painted about a year ago (which I believe you saw) of a Gent and lady at Blackheath both sitting on a Garden settee with a view over the river, for which I had 80. guineas. and in a larger composition the painter should rather aim at making the best picture he can with such a number of figures in such a compass, than oblige himself to such a number of heads, half lengths &c: you see clearly my meaning – when I am asked therefore my price for such pictures I must answer a certain sum – but if left to my self to make the design, I sho.[d] not so much as think of price while composing the Picture, thô I sho.[d] afterwards be obliged to compute by the rule above, which might bring it (on the whole) to more or less than I have askt.[23]

An agreement was reached and in 1743 Highmore produced a double half-length portrait (fig. 23) of Wyndham's sons Wadham (1737–1812) and Henry Penruddocke (1736–1819) and another of Wyndham himself (1743, Yale University Art Gallery) and his brother-in-law Charles Penruddocke (fig. 24). This particular commission from Salisbury was certainly lucrative. In addition to the three male portraits, Highmore was to produce a half-length of Wyndham's wife Arundel (recorded as 1748, possibly a misreading of 1743) and a double portrait of Arundel and her daughter Laetitia (b. 1746).[24] In summary, Highmore's professional association with Warner, Harris and then Wyndham resulted in at least thirteen half-length portraits, five involving two figures, and two 'ancestral' portraits.

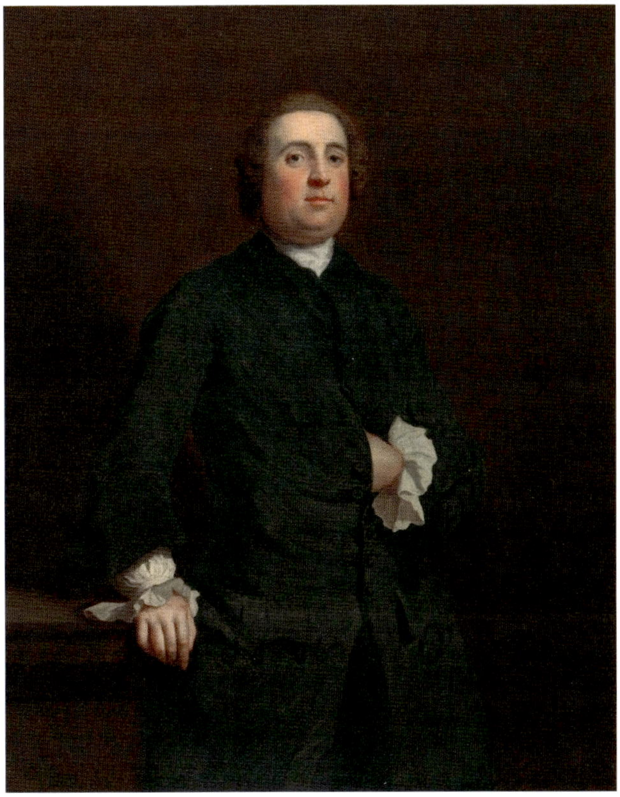

24 Joseph Highmore, *Charles Penruddocke*, 1743, oil on canvas, 127 x 101.3 cm, Yale Center for British Art, Paul Mellon Collection

'HER DEAR BROOD, HER DEAR DELIGHT'

In the same year that he painted Robert and Johanna Warner and their infant, Highmore completed the group portrait *The Family of Sir Eldred Lancelot Lee* (fig. 25). Here all eleven of the main figures, ten Sir Eldred's children, are painted near life size. The only full-length group by Highmore that approaches this in scale and artistic ambition was considered deserving of mention in the *Memoirs*, that is the portrait of 'the Duke of Richmond ... attended by his three Esquires with a perspective view of King Henry the VIIth's Chapel'.[25] No matter how imposing the lost Richmond portrait may have been, *The Lee Family* is without doubt the most ambitious single portrait Highmore ever executed. Since he was an artist who prided himself on painting every element of his portraits himself – shunning the practice of hiring drapery painters, unlike other leading portraitists including Thomas Hudson and Allan Ramsay (1713–1784), declaring to James Harris, 'I do every thing my self, which I believe is not true of one painter in England besides'[26] – the artistic challenge presented by this particular commission was significant.

By the mid 1730s relatively few group portraits were executed on this scale. Sir Eldred (b. 1650) may have commissioned the painting for display at his Shropshire seat, Coton Hall near Alveley. Both he and his brother Thomas were benchers of Lincoln's Inn (their father, Thomas, 1620–1687, had also been a barrister there), providing yet another connection with Highmore's early law career, studio location and, significantly, a direct association with the Harris and Warner families.[27] However, as *The Lee Family* was completed two years after Sir Eldred's death in 1734, the portrait's final appearance, at least, would have been with the agreement of Lee's widow: indeed, and in contrast to the portraits painted for Warner, Harris and Wyndham, it is more likely that it was the widow and mother, Isabella Lee (1690–1767), who was the original commissioner. Analysis of the portrait will bear this out.

For Lady Lee the portrait would have had a variety of functions. In the first instance, it is a visual record of the immediate family members, with the deceased patriarch, Sir Eldred, presented in the background as a partially obscured bust-length portrait, possibly based on a lost painting (attributed to Sir Peter Lely and dated c.1675) that was at one time in the family's possession.[28] The portrait within the portrait operated in the same way as individual pictures in a family gallery and was an appropriate and realistic approach to the representation of the absent or the dead. However, *The Lee Family* also has a metaphysical quality through the inclusion of the infant sibling, Catherine, who had died in 1724 aged only one month, here seen being guided heavenward by an angel.[29]

Regarding ambitious large-scale portrait groups, Highmore clearly used Van Dyck's famed work, *The Family of the 4th Earl of Pembroke* c.1635 (fig. 26) at Wilton House near Salisbury, as one model – a painting described by Carlo Gambarini in 1731 as 'Historical as well as Personal'[30] and one which Highmore could have viewed while visiting his friends and patrons in

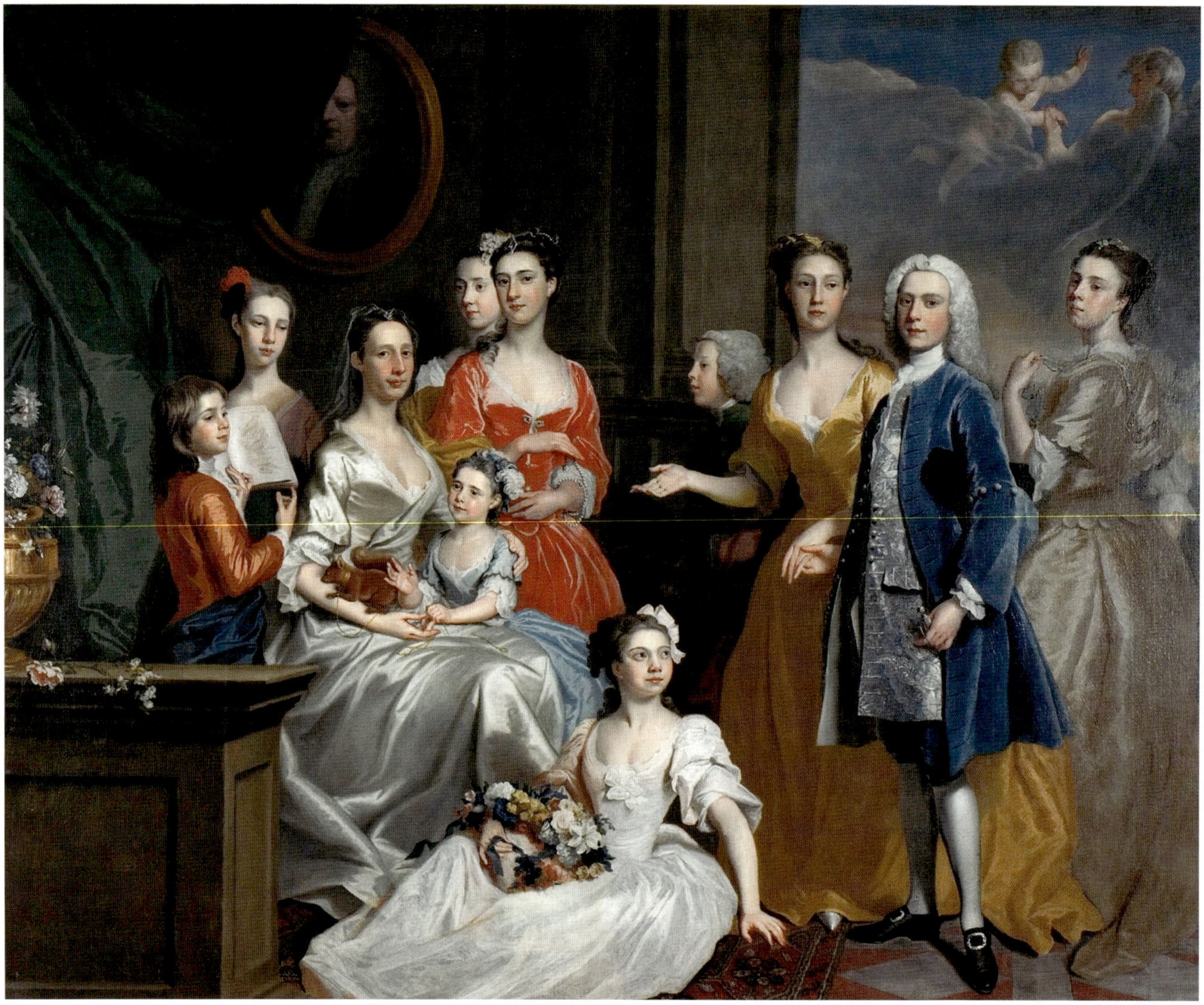

25 Joseph Highmore, *The Family of Sir Eldred Lancelot Lee*, 1736, oil on canvas, 232 x 287 cm, Wolverhampton Art Gallery, Purchased with the assistance of the Victoria and Albert Museum Purchase Grant Fund and Art Fund

Hampshire. Highmore has reproduced, if in reverse, details within the Pembroke painting – the solid architectural backdrop and green draped fabric; the sky and landscape; the device of deceased infants as airborne cherubic figures. Highmore has gathered the Lee family into two distinct groups, one to the left, surrounding the seated Isabella, and a smaller group to the right, gathered around the heir Lancelot (1719–1775); this echoes the groupings in the Pembroke painting. Lancelot is one of three figures looking out, which is likewise seen in the Van Dyck. The middle son Thomas, to the far left in the Highmore painting, stands with his back to the viewer and with a raised right arm: this again refers to the figure in the same position in the Van Dyck. The appearance of the two hounds in the Lee portrait relates to an ancient family obligation to the crown, emphasizing the sense of heritage, tradition and longevity within the painting. At the same time, they evoke the hounds within the Van Dyck portrait. The brother and sister to the right lightly hold hands, in a similar gesture to that linking the couple farthest

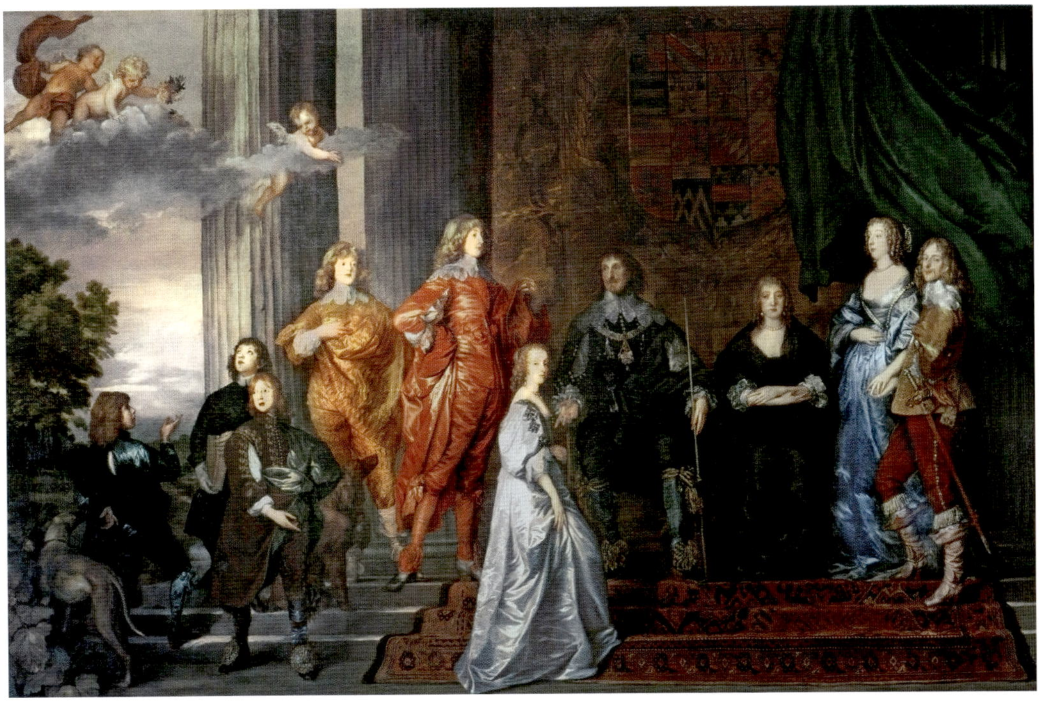

26 Sir Anthony Van Dyck, *Philip Herbert, 4th Earl of Pembroke and his Family*, c.1635, oil on canvas, 279 x 432 cm, Wilton House, Wiltshire

right in the Pembroke painting. Highmore also used similar colours: for example, the red and saffron of the male costumes to the left of the Earl of Pembroke are introduced into the robe and wrap of the eldest daughter, Isabella, standing beside her mother. Meanwhile, the central figure, Matilda, is seated on a Turkey carpet (an item also seen, on a much grander scale, in the Pembroke portrait) but in a more relaxed posture, suggesting a conscious 'loosening' of the rigid standing pose of Van Dyck's central female figure. This introduces a dash of the informality associated with the contemporary 'conversation piece' into what remains, in essence, a formal portrait.

The visual quotations from the Pembroke portrait emphasize the contrast between the portrayals of mothers and motherhood within the two paintings. Traditionally the Pembroke matriarch figure has been identified as the second wife, Lady Anne Clifford, from whom Pembroke was estranged.[31] On this reading, the reality of an unhappy marriage is implied by this figure's isolation, by her morose, uninterested expression and by her black attire, which allows her to sink back into the heraldic tapestry behind. However, in his description of the portrait dated 1731, Gambarini states that the seated figures are '*Philip* Earl of *Pembroke* ... and his Lady, Daughter to the Earl of Oxford, with their five Sons and one Daughter',[32] that is, Pembroke's deceased first wife, Lady Susan de Vere, the mother of the Pembroke children. Her inclusion means the family line – the dead as well as the living – are represented and she is appropriately portrayed in an almost shadowy or otherworldly manner. The accompanying dark-toned costume of the still living husband seems to signal that the older generation will soon be completely eclipsed by the next, indicated by the vibrant colours of the assembled children and spouses.

In contrast to Anne/Susan, Isabella Lee is not presented as a distant or declining force. She is seated and 'raised' like her seventeenth-century predecessor, but is wearing virtuous white rather than funereal

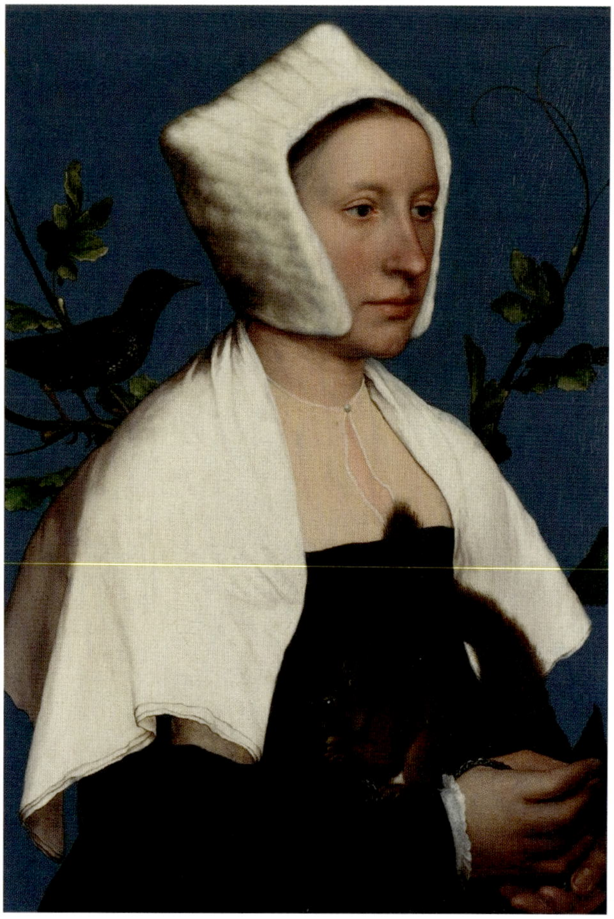

27 Hans Holbein the Younger, *Lady with a Squirrel and a Starling*, c.1526–28, oil on oak, 56 x 38.8 cm, The National Gallery, London

black. In fact, despite the relatively recent loss of her husband, here she has not been specifically defined in the role of widow. Far from fading into the subdued tones of the scenery behind her, she sits as a prominent symbol of the chaste wife and fertile mother, the epitome of spiritual purity and natural fecundity.

For many years it was supposed that the portrait had been commissioned to commemorate the imminent departure of Lancelot to manage the family's foreign commercial interests and property. The key evidence for this interpretation is the book held up by Thomas, identifiable as *Ornithologiae Libri Tres* by Francis Willughby (London, 1676), which is opened to a page illustrating parrots native to Africa, Indonesia and South America.[33] However, there is no documentation explaining how this interpretation emerged.[34] On the contrary, as far as it can be established, Sir Eldred's estates did not extend beyond England and he intended his heir to enter, or at least receive training in, his own profession at Lincoln's Inn.[35] In reality, the direct connection to foreign trade springs from Isabella, whose uncle, Sir Richard Gough (d. 1727/28), a close associate of the prominent and influential City merchant Sir John Houblon, acquired a fortune through trading speculations in East India and China.[36] Three of Isabella's brothers also had close associations with the East India Company.[37] Therefore the parrot illustration is a signal of the status and wealth of Isabella's family, the Goughs. This union of two powerful families – embodied by the Lee children – is then emphatically stated in the shield, located at the top centre of the ornately carved frame, which combines the arms of Lee and Gough.

The portrait, in general, represents the shift in family circumstances after Sir Eldred's death in 1734. But, given that Lancelot entered Lincoln's Inn on 6 June 1735 (along with his brother Harry, seen centre back), it is this later event that most likely inspired the commission and was the means through which the Lees came into contact with the artist – establishing a further association between the Lee, Warner and Harris families.[38] Yet, if these circumstances explain why Lancelot provides one focal point within the portrait, it is important to recognize that the other focal point is Isabella herself. She sits directly below the portrait of her dead husband, the 'absent' patriarch whom she had married in 1713, and it is on her arm that the family's heraldic symbol, a collared and chained red squirrel, rests. This precise juxtaposition between Isabella, the Lee's heraldic animal and the illustration of a bird mimics Hans Holbein's *Lady with a Squirrel and a Starling* of about 1526–28 (fig. 27), offering an early artistic model and further pedigree to the composition and its subject.[39] As one of only two seated figures, and the only one raised on a step, Isabella is by ancient social custom the most important figure in the group. Symbolically and physically, Sir Eldred's family line and lineage continues through Isabella, and, at this time, and in his absence, it is through her alone that the line will continue to be supported and nurtured. Isabella was her husband's executrix and, according to his will, she had the 'use of all my goods ... for life, and after that to my son Lancelot if he marry in his mothers lifetime and with her consent'.[40] Lancelot was indeed Sir Eldred's heir and Highmore's depiction of him acknowledges this. But at seventeen he had not yet come of age.

To emphasize her continued high status, indeed dominance, all of Isabella's children are already gathered around her, are indicating towards her, or are in the process of moving towards her. She is the epicentre of the portrait and by extension the family, and her children naturally gravitate to and around her. This movement from right to left is initially signalled by the right hand of Dorothy, the daughter centrally placed and dressed in a saffron gown.[41] Through this prominent, isolated gesture, the sister invites her brother to move towards their mother – an action Lancelot is in the process of making, as shown by the precise shift of weight to his right leg and the almost balletic lift of his left foot. In support of the elder son's new public role and imminent departure to London, he is shown with a black hat tucked under his arm and a sword by his side. The setting that Highmore has created for this narrative is a monumental stone structure that opens out to the elements and to the park landscape beyond, providing a perfect stage for this symbolic movement between the exterior and the interior, the public and the private.

The general sense of movement towards Isabella is also shown in the figure of the daughter, Mary, standing to the far right. Prior to the moment captured, she appears to have been watching her infant sister being raised to heaven, while absently holding or playing with her gauze headdress. Highmore has painted her just after she has turned back and prior to her joining her living siblings. The curve of her right hand and arm, as well as her pose, mirrors and therefore balances the pose of her brother standing to the far left. The gathering momentum from right to left suggests that, in a few moments' time, all the figures will be brought securely within the solid stone structure and directly under the protective eye of Sir Eldred. Despite the painting's formality, the figures seem at ease within this setting. This image presents the Lee family as a well-ordered but not rigid household and therefore, by extension, genteel, good-mannered and dutiful citizens – a description which chimes with Highmore's later observation, 'much of the general good of society depending on the wise and just government of families'.[42]

As is suggested by the self-conscious symbolism within the portrait – which includes the family jewellery held up by the eldest daughter, Isabella – the Lee family were very mindful of a lineage which, according to family tradition, combined Saxon and Norman stock, and of a gentrified existence that they had scrupulously maintained for seven centuries. Even the name 'Lancelot' conjures up an ancient, chivalric past. The sense of pride in this lineage is nicely captured in a long letter concerning the family's history written by Lancelot in 1745:

> It is very extraordinary that any family, considering the great revolutions that have so frequently happened in England, should remain for nearly 700 years in the same state which our family has done. The last two or three generations must certainly have been very frugal, or they could not have preserved the estate. Variety of wives and a large number of daughters are a very heavy weight upon land, and can only be balanced by very prudent management. The estate has been increased only in proportion to the value of money. By this may very fairly be collected that we are not an avaricious people.[43]

Writing in the May of 1745, Lancelot had no idea that Britain was within months of plunging into a yet another period of political and social turmoil – the '45 Jacobite Rebellion. That aside, Highmore's portrait signifies the steadiness and durability, as well as ancient descent, of the Lee dynasty.

In her article on representations of the dead within eighteenth-century family portraiture, Kate Retford has explored the symbolism within *The Lee Family*, particularly the contrast in which the deceased father, in the oval portrait, and the infant daughter, as 'putto', have been portrayed.[44] She rightly observes, as a general rule, that the use of a portrait within a portrait was 'most popularly employed ... as a means of dealing with the untimely death of a pater familias'.[45] However, this explanation is less compelling in relation to the Lee family, given that Sir Eldred was sixty-four years old when he married Isabella (then twenty-three) in 1713 and therefore his death twenty-one years later must have been far from unexpected. Meanwhile, in a period in which, in urban environments, between one fifth and one quarter of live births died before the age of two, the death of an infant was, tragically, all too common. Isabella herself was the second youngest of sixteen children, five of whom died in infancy.[46] It is extraordinary, then, that Isabella and Sir Eldred succeeded in producing ten healthy children (with no multiple births) within two decades of marriage.

In the light of this, it could be argued that it is the celebration of life, conjugal love, fecundity and, ultimately, motherhood, that is the primary focus of the portrait. This is supported by Isabella's choice of dress, no more than two years after her husband's death – an oyster-white gown and white veil, rather than a widow's weeds. In fact white is Highmore's favoured colour for the mothers in his mother-and-child portraits. Meanwhile, the assembly of bright hues surrounding the luminous white of Isabella's robe creates a remarkably intense effect. In their respective colours – vermilion-red, saffron, blue, green, pink, white and copper – the children gather around their mother rather like a festoon or garland of rich and precious flowers. This is echoed by the presence of the garland held by the seated Matilda, which contains colours mirrored in the children's costumes.

The portrait could therefore be seen as an allegory of the bounty of nature. Certainly Highmore would have been fully aware of the use of flowers and cultivated gardens as metaphors of love, marriage and parenthood. Considering his particular interest in Rubens, the paintings *Rubens and Isabella Brant in the Honeysuckle Bower* (as described in 1732 at the Elector

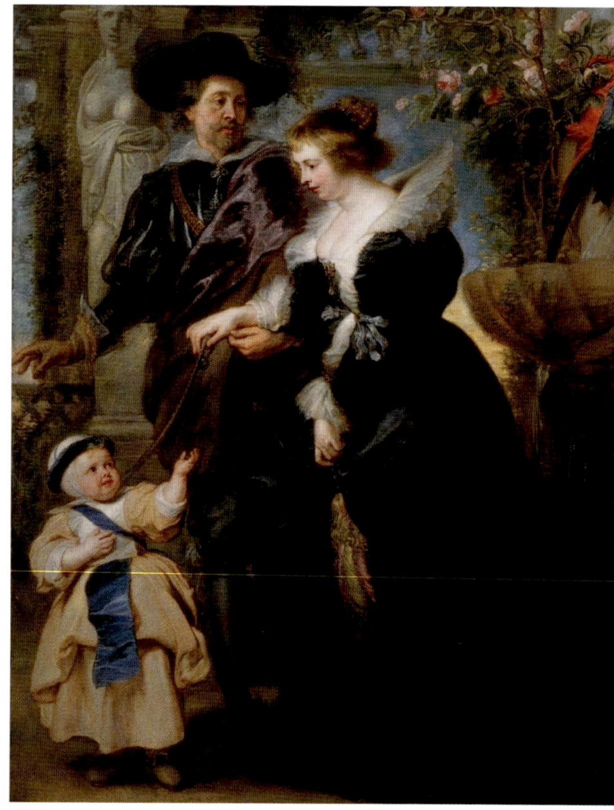

28 Sir Peter Paul Rubens, *The Artist, his Wife Hélène Fourment and their Son Frans*, c.1635, oil on wood, 203.8 x 158.1 cm, The Metropolitan Museum of Art, New York, Gift of Mr. and Mrs. Charles Wrightsman, in honor of Sir John Pope-Hennessy, 1981

Palatine's Gallery, Düsseldorf), *Rubens, his Wife Hélène Fourment and their Son Frans* (from 1722 to 1883 in the Marlborough collection at Blenheim Palace; fig. 28) and his monumental allegory of the stages of courtship and marriage *The Garden of Love* (prime version, Museo del Prado, Madrid; fig. 29) would all have served as powerful visual examples.[47] In the first and second paintings, the plants, such as the honeysuckle, are symbolic of fertility within marriage and therefore signal the particular purpose of each portrait – in the first the hope of children, in the second the realisation of that hope. Highmore's introduction of a jasmine shrub – an evergreen plant that represents virtue –into his portrait of his own wife and children (see fig. 15) is an earlier example of his use of such floral symbolism within family-group portraits.

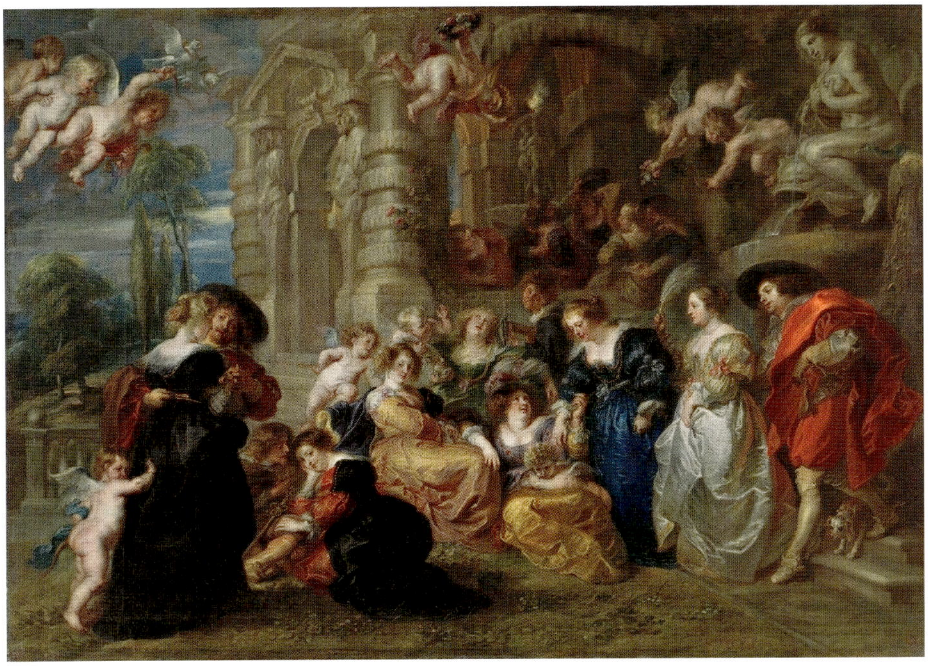

29 Sir Peter Paul Rubens, *The Garden of Love*, c.1633, oil on canvas, 199 x 286 cm, Museo Nacional del Prado, Madrid

Meanwhile from Rubens's *Garden of Love* (see fig. 29), a composition dominated by women, the male figure encouraging the young female to move towards the assembly, and the central pair of women, one of whom leans on her companion's lap, are echoed in Highmore's own female-dominated painting. Further, the 'garden', presided over by the nursing Venus and the Graces, is a terrace set out before a monumental stone structure and steps, in fact Rubens's own house in Antwerp. The natural world, in the form of landscape and trees, is contained within the top left of the painting, allowing the rich colours – red, white, saffron, blue and green – to be introduced through the costumes of the gathering lovers, who become the cultivated ornaments of this metaphorical garden. Above them hover *amorini*. All these motifs are found in the Lee family portrait.

The floral symbolism in *The Lee Family* continues in a different form through an arrangement in the copper vase on the stone plinth to the far left. This small 'still life' appears to be modelled on seventeenth-century Netherlandish flower paintings. Some of the blooms have tumbled on to the plinth, suggesting that these flowers have begun to droop and wither in the style of a *vanitas*, a reminder of the fleeting nature of youth, beauty and ultimately life itself. A similar motif can be seen in *'John Rich and Family'* (see fig. 21): in this instance a basket of fruit is resting on an identical stone plinth. The contrast between the wilting flowers, representing a future state of decay, and the vibrant garland that lies on Matilda's lap hints that the garland serves as a symbol of the present, the here and now, rather than the future or the past.

In addition, as seen in history paintings depicting scenes as varied as classical triumphs and ancient or pagan festivals, the garland that Matilda holds could soon be used to adorn someone or something – the hero, god or goddess – in celebration of a recent deed or event, or in honour of their elevated status. As I have observed, Highmore owned and copied a version of Rubens's *Venus Genetrix* (fig. 30) depicting a term, representing the Great Mother Nature, adorned with a ripe garland of fruit and crowned with flowers

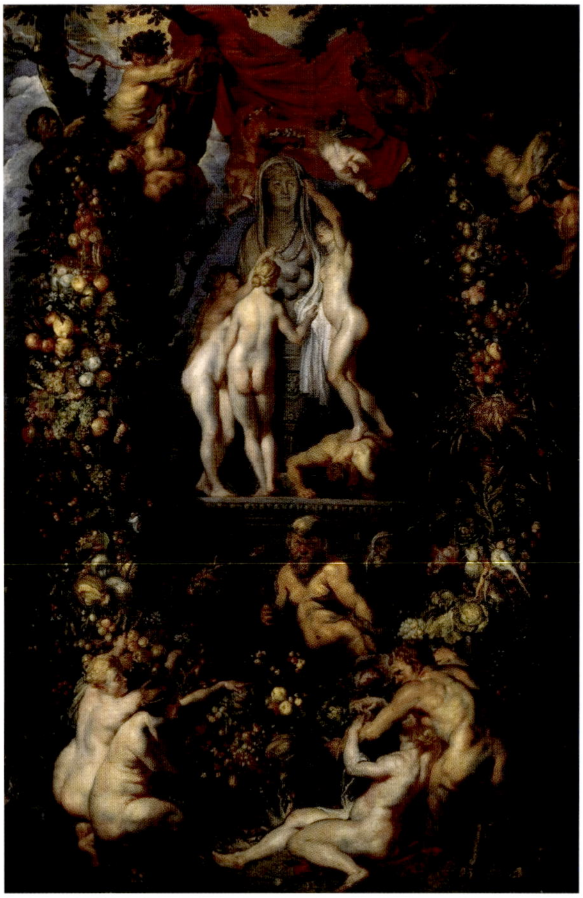

30 Sir Peter Paul Rubens and Jan Brueghel I, *Venus Genetrix*, c.1615, oil on panel, 106.7 x 72.4 cm, Kelvingrove Art Gallery and Museum, Glasgow

by amorini. Therefore Highmore's floral imagery, coupled with the presence of her children, may signify Isabella's personification of the Mother Goddess or Nature.[48] Highmore was to use the motif of a garland in the portrait of Elizabeth Lee (the daughter here seen leaning on her mother's knee) in 1755, the year of her marriage to William Waller, barrister of Lincoln's Inn (also Wolverhampton Art Gallery). In this later instance, the garland might represent a tribute by Elizabeth to the god of marriage feasts, Hymen, for a successful and fruitful union. Highmore again used the garland in the portrait, *Mrs Elizabeth Birch and her daughter* of 1741 (fig. 31). The young daughter, like a bacchic nymph or 'child of nature', wears a posy of buds in her hair and is holding up the garland to adorn her mother. Similarly in the Highmore family portrait (see fig. 15), the daughter Susanna is playfully dressed as an infant goddess Flora, wearing a floral coronet and offering roses and jasmine to her brother. As Anthony is holding the instruments of his future trade as a draughtsman, perhaps this portrait signifies the son's formal or informal apprenticeship into his father's profession.

In this sense, the female figures in the Lee portrait, and particularly Matilda, may be assuming the role of handmaidens, or perhaps of the Graces. However, by placing Matilda between her mother and brother, Highmore allows for two scenarios and two roles for the garland. It may soon adorn the mother as a symbol of her marriage and motherhood. However, Matilda is also looking back and up at her elder brother. Therefore the garland may be intended for him: a symbol of his newly elevated position within the family and recent entry into his father's profession, coupled with the longed-for hope of another fruitful marriage that will continue the Lee family line.

There is also, finally, the potential to make an association between Isabella and the most celebrated Christian mother figure of all, the Virgin Mary. Highmore's use of blue and white in the dress of mothers and their children, as already suggested, refers to the traditional colour of the Madonna: the high value, semi-precious lapis lazuli pigment being reserved for the Mother of God. Of greater significance, in this instance, are Rubens's various paintings of the Virgin and Child, framed by a burgeoning garland of brightly coloured flowers and cherubs. Highmore would have seen a version at the Elector Palatine's Gallery at Düsseldorf in 1732 (now Alte Pinakotek, Munich).

The presence of the parrot motif in *The Lee Family*, cleverly introduced through the book illustration held up by Thomas, does not simply represent earthly possessions and a source of family status and wealth. As a device associated with the Virgin Mary, the parrot can be seen here to symbolise the purity and self-sacrifice of a mother's love.[49] Rubens reflected such multi-layered symbolism in images of the Holy Family and in his self-portrait with his second wife and child from the 1630s (see above). In turn, and in the same

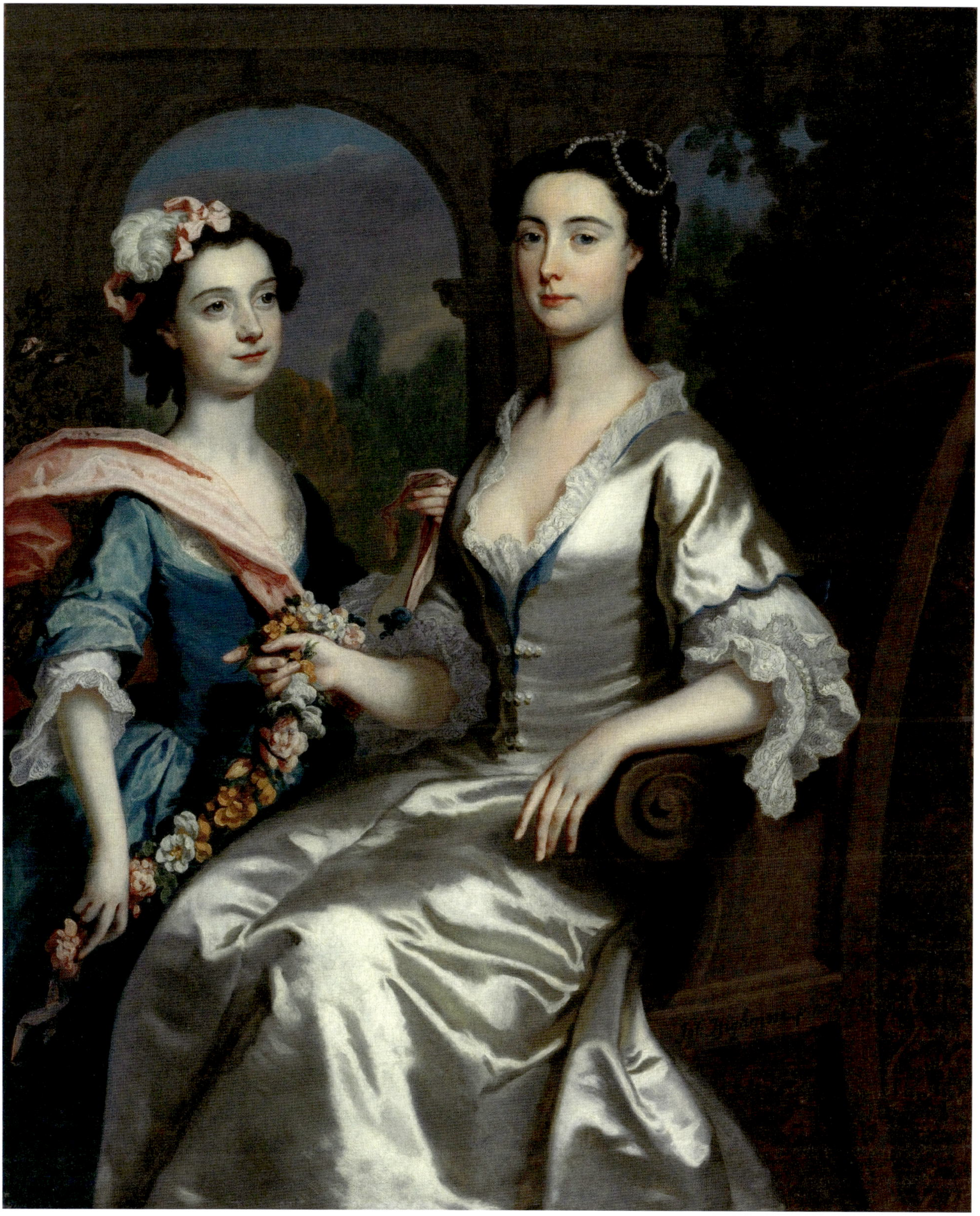

31 Joseph Highmore, *Mrs Elizabeth Birch and her Daughter*, 1741,
oil on canvas, 119.1 x 97.2 cm, The Fitzwilliam Museum, Cambridge

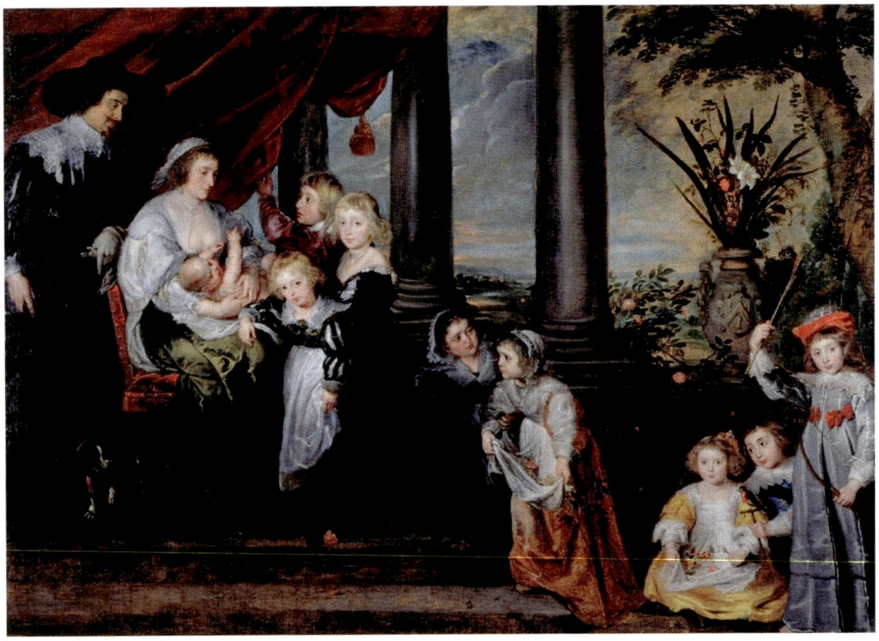

32 Attributed to Sir Peter Paul Rubens, *The Family of Sir Balthazar Gerbier*, c.1629–41, oil on canvas, 217.2 x 310 cm, The British Royal Collection

context, Highmore had used this particular symbol in his 1731 portrait of mother and infant, *Mrs Sharpe and her Child* (see fig. 97), possibly the same 'Mrs. Sharpe' named as the artist's cousin in his will.[50] Intriguingly, the association of the parrot with Mary and the birth of Jesus came, originally, from a story relating to the Roman Emperor Augustus Caesar. After his victory over Mark Antony at Actium, Octavian (later styled Emperor Augustus) was greeted by a parrot with the phrase 'Ave Caesar', an omen of his future greatness.[51] This in turn became a coded prophecy of the archangel Gabriel's greeting to Mary 'Ave Maria' or 'Hail Mary' (the feast of the Annunciation). Therefore, in this single motif, Highmore succeeds in combining the Gough family's trading links with Isabella's maternal love and even to the future greatness of the Lee family's own young 'Caesar', Lancelot.

In fact many of the compositional structures and motifs described above – the architectural setting, the seated and raised mother, the 'parade' of children (including a seated 'Matilda' figure), the parrot, the dog, the plinth, the vase of flowers, the floral offerings – can be found in the Rubens studio portrait of *The Family of Sir Balthasar Gerbier* (fig. 32), a work considered in the mid eighteenth century to be by either Rubens or Van Dyck and in 1749 purchased from an unidentified collection in Flanders for Frederick Louis, Prince of Wales.[52] If in Flanders in 1732, then this would explain the strong visual connections to Highmore's portrait, although it is also true that Rubens constantly reused such motifs and postures from his own paintings. Either way, *The Lee Family* is a fusion of elements predominantly, but not exclusively, from works by Rubens and Van Dyck, which have been reconfigured, repurposed and updated for a modern English family.

'ALL THINGS DECAY IN TIME'

Despite the portrait's celebration of life, love and youth, death is also present. It is initially signalled by the posthumous representation of the father and infant daughter and then emphasized by the allegorical still-life *vanitas*, which acts as the augury of death and decay for everyone depicted. The representation of the infant, who unlike Sir Eldred had died twelve years prior to the creation of the portrait, is a conscious reference to the idea of the soul's separation from the body at death. In the contemporary writings of Highmore's friend and theological mentor Dr Isaac Watts, some solace is offered to mourners by encouraging them to focus on the joy experienced by the departed's soul in heaven, or 'those upper and brighter Regions, than to be ever dwelling upon the dark Prospect, and fixing our Eyes upon Death, and Dust, and the Grave'.[53] He also describes how the separated body is kept imprisoned on earth within the grave by 'Death', but that death is only the temporary custodian. For, Watts continues, as promised through Christ's crucifixion and resurrection, on the Day of Judgment death will be conquered and the body will finally be released to join the soul.[54] The arrangement of the Lee family is symbolic of the separation between the living (below) and the dead (above), but coupled with the hope of the family's future reunion in heaven. Little Catherine's presence, in her physical, earthly form as she moves towards heaven, suggests that we are witnessing a premonition of the reunion of her body with her soul. This vision brings great comfort to her mother and family, while, at the same time, indicating their own future state on earth and then in heaven.

If the portrait's compositional models and symbolism, as set out here, are taken together, the painting can also be seen as a reflection on the cycle of life and death – the transient nature of the former and the inevitability of the latter – coupled with the process of renewal. The representation of the father and daughter, offering a dramatic contrast in their ages at death, hints at the arbitrariness of this cycle. If Isaac Watts offered comfort in his concept of heaven and the deceased, their current and future state, then this portrait, too, offers consolation in its layered references to the onward movement of time, even as it suspends it. Within the painting there is a constant play, back and forth, between 'reality' and allegory, and within time itself: we see an infant, who died over a decade before the portrait was conceived, together with a man who died more recently and in his mid eighties, yet is represented here in middle age. As regards the patron, the portrait is as much a reflection of Isabella's personal attitude towards motherhood and family – the private joy and pain she derives from them – as it is a statement of heritage and dynastic continuity. And, as an allegory on life *and* death, the picture may have celebrated literary as well as theological and visual models.

In 1715 the poet John Hughes sent a copy of his most recent publication to Sir Godfrey Kneller observing in the covering letter, 'Knowing how great an admirer you are of Rubens, and of his genius for allegorical painting, I could not avoid thinking of you when I undertook to publish Spenser, who had the same genius with Rubens, and is the most painter-like poet'.[55] This publication was the first illustrated edition of the complete works of the Elizabethan poet Edmund Spenser, with designs by Kneller's fellow academy director, Louis du Guernier (1677–1716). In his response, Kneller thanks Hughes for 'the most acceptable present of Mr Spencer's worcks [sic]'.[56] A volume was included in Kneller's Kit-Cat portrait of Lord Somers, to whom Hughes had dedicated his project. Among the two hundred subscribers are listed William Cheselden, James Thornhill and Jonathan Richardson, which, with the inclusion of Kneller and Du Guernier, establishes a connection between Hughes's publication and directors or prominent members of the Great Queen Street Academy during Highmore's membership. In 1731 another stalwart of the academy, George Vertue, was himself compiling a life of the poet, whom he describes as 'that Famous Poet. and our Second Chaucer'.[57] On a fundamental level, the support given to Hughes's publication is an example of the broader intellectual interests and associations encouraged within the early London art academies. In fact Highmore may well have been introduced to the poet from a very early age, given that Spenser was a famous 'old boy' of Highmore's school, Merchant Taylors'.

I have established elsewhere that Newtonian imagery, as epitomized by Hughes's metaphysical poem 'The Ecstasy', was introduced into Highmore's 'double' portrait of the renowned natural philosopher Sir Isaac

Newton and the ivory carver David Le Marchand, therefore establishing an early link not only between Hughes and Highmore but between the symbolism within Hughes's publications and its selective use by the painter in his portraits.[58] This association can be confirmed through the presence of Highmore's early patrons and the commissioners of the Le Marchand portrait, Mathew and Moses Raper, as subscribers to Hughes's *Works of Spenser*. In his letter to Kneller, quoted above, Hughes makes a direct correlation between Kneller and Rubens and, through allegorical painting and poetry, between Rubens and Spenser – associations that would have been of great interest to the younger artist. Further, John Hughes was the brother-in-law of Highmore's close friend William Duncombe (father of Highmore's son-in-law, John). In 1735, Duncombe published a two-volume collection of Hughes's poems, to which Highmore had subscribed, and in which Duncombe refers to Hughes's edition 'of the Works of our famous Poet Mr. *Edmund Spenser*'.[59]

Hughes, described in *The Cambridge Companion to Spenser* as 'one of Spenser studies' founding figures',[60] observes in his introductory 'Essay on Allegorical Poetry' that allegory is 'a kind of Poetical Picture; or Hieroglyphick' and later, 'The Resemblance which has been so often observ'd in general between Poetry and Painting, is yet more particular in Allegory; which, as I said before, is a kind of Picture in Poetry'.[61] Further on, Hughes highlights one of Rubens's paintings from the Marie des Médicis cycle as a pre-eminent example of visual allegory.[62] This was the series that Highmore would spend many hours studying in Paris just prior to the Lee portrait commission. Spenser's allegories – although considered obscure by many – were beginning to gain value and prominence, not only as prime examples of literary invention but as a way of transferring complex ideas concerning the human condition.[63] For an accomplished artist, according to Jonathan Richardson, such erudition was vital: 'What I have hitherto said will be of little Use to him who does not *Fill and Supply his Mind with Noble Images*. A Painter should therefore read the Best Books, such as *Homer, Milton, Virgil, Spencer, Thucydides, Livy, Plutarch*, &c.'[64] Clearly, familiarity with Spenser was seen as part of the broader development of literary knowledge and understanding, that, in turn, stimulated a sophistication in manner and invention within an artist's practice. Such levels of sophistication were as appropriate here in *The Lee Family*, a portrait that strove to be, in Gambarini's words, 'Historical as well as Personal', as they would be for subject or history painting.

In his introductory remarks on *The Faerie Queene*, Hughes highlighted a particular passage from Spenser's epic poem as one of the poet's great allegorical inventions.[65] It appears within the description of 'The Garden of Adonis', where exists 'all the goodly Flowers/ Wherewith Dame Nature doth her beautify', 'the first Seminary/Of all things, that are born to live and die' and 'the endless Progeny/Of all the Weeds, that bud and blossom there'.[66] This passage can be seen as a blending of the symbolism associated with motherhood, nature and flora (discussed above). The Lee children represent the 'garden' established and nurtured through the union of Isabella and Sir Eldred and who, as symbolized by their vivid-coloured costumes, 'bud and blossom'. Yet, as Spenser continues and Highmore's imagery, in turn, sets out, they are 'born to live and die'. Spenser's 'endless Progeny', that is the countless generations that will derive from these 'weeds', alludes to ancestry and more specifically to dynastic continuation – one of the preoccupations of the Lee family portrait.

As described by Hughes, 'The Figure of Time walking in this Garden, spoiling the Beauty of it, and cutting down the Flowers, is a very fine and significant Allegory'.[67] This particular allegory is a reminder that, in order to achieve dynastic renewal, the living must die. Turning to the Lee portrait, it is Sir Eldred's death that allows Lancelot to realise his destiny. The language used by Spenser conjures up a pitiless, undiscerning figure, relentlessly and randomly destroying all 'the flowring Herbs and goodly things ... both Leaves and Buds without regard,/ Ne ever pity may relent his Malice hard.'[68] This provides a context within which the death of Sir Eldred and his infant daughter can be explained and accommodated – not only the arbitrariness of death, but its presence even in the most perfect of circumstances. Finally, Spenser's 'great Mother *Venus*' or 'Dame Nature', although lamenting the process and 'The Loss of her dear Brood, her dear Delight' – as she is the creator of life, death is anathema to her – nonetheless she takes some comfort in the certainty that 'all that lives is subject to that Law:/ All things decay in time, and to their end do draw'.[69]

Similarly Isabella's expression of dignified sadness and her protective gesture towards her youngest child suggest that the pleasure she draws from her living children has been tempered by the loss of her little daughter. She has, after all, and some twelve years after the death, requested Catherine's symbolic inclusion as a 'living' entity. And this in stark contrast to the representation of her husband. Through the correspondence with James Harris, we have seen how Highmore guided his client through the options available for their portraits. It can be imagined that some, if not all, of his ideas for this portrait, in fulfilment of her own vision for it, must have been explained and discussed with Isabella. At the same time she surely allowed him creative freedom. Perhaps here Highmore was, as he had written to James Harris, 'left to my self to make the design' and, with money no object, 'I sho.[d] not so much as think of price while composing the Picture'. Either way, Highmore has not stressed one particular narrative or model, nor has he created a thoroughgoing visual allegory, as can be seen in Rubens's Marie des Médicis cycle. This is first and foremost a portrait of a modern family, but one with a strong sense of maternal, familial and dynastic ties, which Highmore has chosen to reflect through a deep and complex layering of explicit and implicit symbolism and allegory.

'FRIEND AND LOVER'

As discussed earlier, the group portrait *The Vigor Family* (fig. 33) is a very rare example of a family piece or 'conversation' by Highmore – a fact that is at complete odds with his reputation for such portraits both during his lifetime and at his death. The Vigor group is located within an aristocratic-style interior, with stone walls, pillars and a distinctive red and white chequered floor – all demonstrating Highmore's ability in the use of perspective. The portrait depicts five figures: Jane Vigor (1699–1783), who is seated to the far left; her third husband, the Quaker merchant William Vigor (d.1767), who is standing to the right and indicates towards her; his brother Joseph, who is standing centrally; seated before him, his wife Ann, who pauses at her task and turns to look at Jane; and then seated to her left, someone who can be identified as John Penn (1700–1746), son of William Penn the founder of Pennsylvania and a Vigor family friend. In the same year Highmore painted individual portraits of John and his brothers, William and Thomas, and John's portrait is clearly the source of his image within the Vigor family group.[70] John was the only Penn child to be born in the New World (in Philadelphia), although raised in Bristol, and was known within his family as 'The American'.[71]

If a single event acted as the spur for the commissioning of a group portrait, perhaps John Penn's visit to Highmore's studio, it is clear through the placing of figures, their gestures, and the objects introduced into the painting, that other events or associations are also being celebrated. Jane had spent many years in Russia with her first husband, Thomas Ward (d. 1731), the British consul general to the Russian Imperial Court, and then her second husband, Claudius Rondeau, who succeeded Thomas as consul general. There is a hint that Jane and Claudius were expecting a child while in St Petersburg. In 1733 Jane recalls that a Russian nobleman visited her the day after she 'was brought to bed' and, after paying his compliments, 'gave me a ducat, which he could not omit, as they fancy either the woman or the child will die, if they did not do it. This', she continues 'would have diverted me, if I had not been more dead than alive at that time.' She describes convalescing for three months and, as there is no mention of a child, it must be presumed that the infant was still-born or died soon after. The experience must have been terrible. Jane herself admitted, at the time, 'as this is the first, I should be horribly frighted if I was to find myself in the same condition again'.[72] There is no mention of children from any of her marriages,

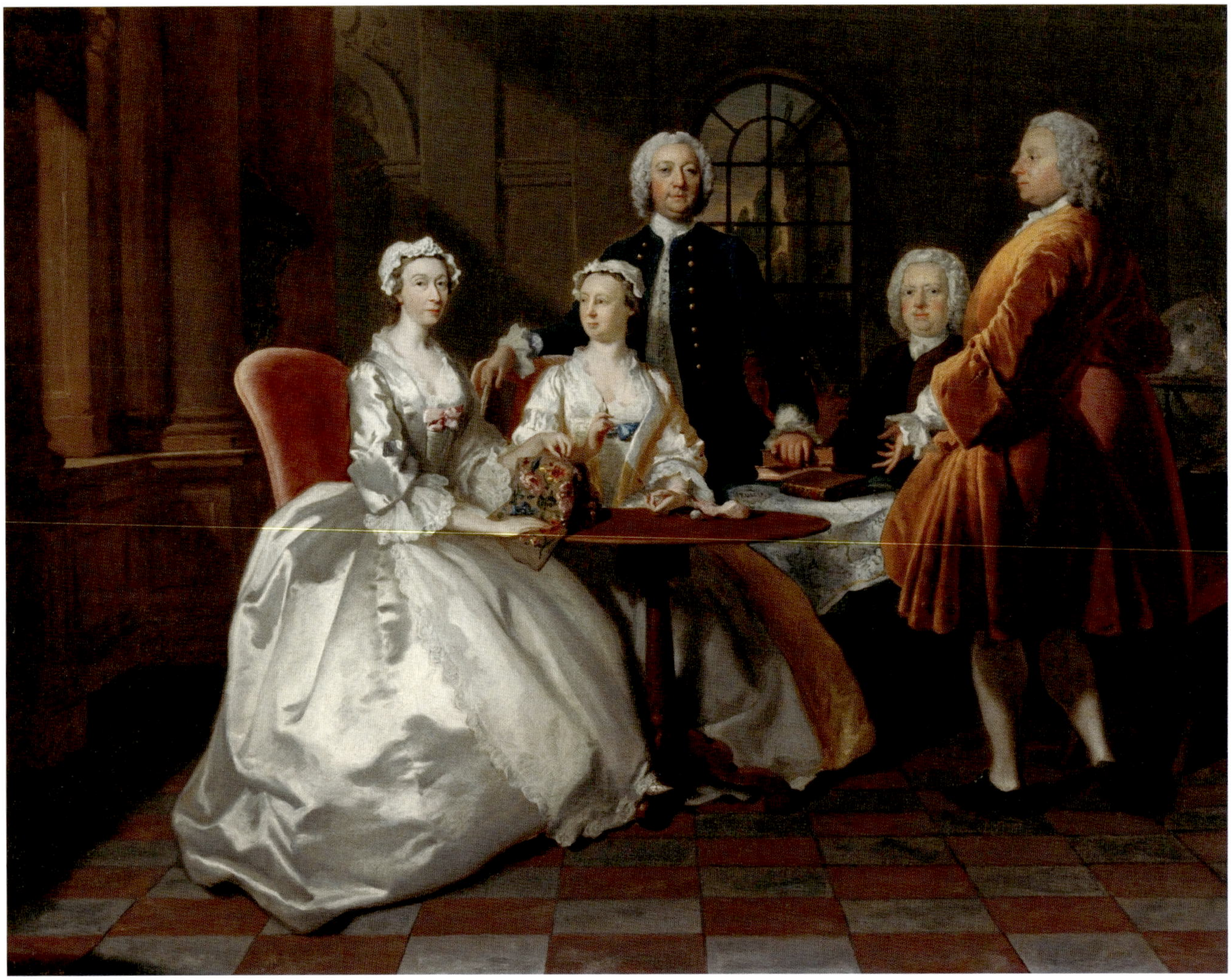

33 Joseph Highmore, *The Vigor Family*, 1744, oil on canvas, 76.2 x 99.1 cm, Victoria and Albert Museum, London

as the absence of offspring in the Vigor group portrait appears to confirm.

The association between the women and needlework, in particular the exquisite floral embroidery that Jane is holding up (examples can be seen at the Victoria and Albert Museum) might at first glance indicate modest domestic industry – also represented by Jane's apron – which is, at the same time, suggestive of leisure.[73] Yet, while in Russia, this accomplishment was the means by which an Englishwoman, with little Russian but some French (the language of the court) could not only develop a camaraderie, even intimacy, with high-ranking Russian aristocrats, but with Tzarina Anna (b. 1693) herself. Jane recounts occasions when, while embroidering with Countess Biron in her apartment adjoining those of the Tzarina (Count Biron was Anna's chief advisor and lover), the Tzarina, who ruled the Russian Empire in her own right, 'sometimes sits down at the same frame, and works with us'. Jane observes that such moments of intimacy were invaluable to her husband's status and business at court, while, on a personal level, allowing Jane to see the Tzarina in a very different light, having 'great pleasure in observing so much humanity in one who has such despotic power'.[74] Jane's embroidery therefore holds a very particular significance, well beyond the domestic. The presence of Ann as Jane's companion in the embroidering process suggests that she has assumed the role of Countess Biron or perhaps, given the happenstance of her name, Tsarina Anna. There is a paradox, therefore, and some humour – an in-joke – in this representation of what was considered, traditionally, a modest domestic female accomplishment.

In her letters from St Petersburg, later published to great acclaim, Jane also describes the *dacha*, a plain, wooden country house, rented by the couple, in which she wittily describes them spending half the week in humble, rustic bliss. The house 'as it is rural without … is rural within', 'no art or cultivation' displayed, but modestly furnished with white calico, rush chairs and delftware. Cows and sheep amble around it, occasionally wandering up to the open windows. 'One parlour,' Jane writes, 'is furnished with books and maps; those, and my frame for embroidery, are the only things that make it differ from a farm.' Jane concludes the description of their Russian idyll with a poignant comment on her husband Claudius: 'I have in him the confidence of friendship and the tenderness of love; and while heaven spares me this friend and lover, I shall be happy in all vicissitudes of fortune'.[75]

This was written in 1734. Five years later, Claudius had died and Jane was returning to England a widow twice over. In response, Tzarina Anna, 'having particular benevolence towards the said Widow for her good deserts, and consequently taking a share in her welfare [and] desirous on Our side any way to promote it', wrote to her 'brother' King George II 'to recommend her to your Majesty's most high Protection in the best manner, requesting your Majesty as a friend and Sister to show the said Widow in her supplication, Your Royal Favour to her advantage and Consolation, in the melancholy station she is in'.[76] This displays extraordinary compassion and attention towards a woman in distress, particularly notable from one with 'despotic power', and reveals the high esteem in which Jane was held by the Tzarina. The translator himself notes that 'the Original was sign'd with Her Imp[eria]l M[a]jes[t]ys owne hand'.

Jane was escorted home by William Vigor and they married in 1740.[77] The globe to the right of the Vigor group portrait and the map of Russia on the table in front of John Penn – to which Vigor is also indicating as he gestures to his wife – confirms the role that travel, and Russia in particular, has played in their introduction and marriage. Yet – recalling the descriptions of the *dacha* – the maps and the embroidery also act as a subtle reminder of Jane's life prior to her meeting William and therefore another relationship, the loss of which she must have continued to mourn, given her heartfelt (and later public) declaration regarding Claudius, her friend and lover.

The positioning of William Vigor, with his back to the viewer, while looking at and gesturing towards his wife, establishes that she is the key figure within the portrait. Ann's glance towards her sister-in-law supports this. Indeed, the manner in which William is posed – facing into the composition and gazing across it, rather than presenting himself to and looking out at the viewer of the painting – establishes his desire to be shown in a secondary role to his wife. Jane is placed in the same location within the portrait and in the same position and posture as Isabella Lee and, as echoed in this earlier family image, figures within the Vigor portrait are facing or indicating towards her. However, unlike *The Lee Family*, all the figures in the Vigor portrait are middle aged; Jane is now 45 years old (incidentally the same age as Isabella Lee in the earlier portrait). It can therefore be viewed as representing an alternative or parallel life-model for a middling-sort female and one as potentially fulfilling as that represented by Isabella and her children – a celebration of mature love, support and partnership between men and women and, more broadly, the companionship and friendship of equals.

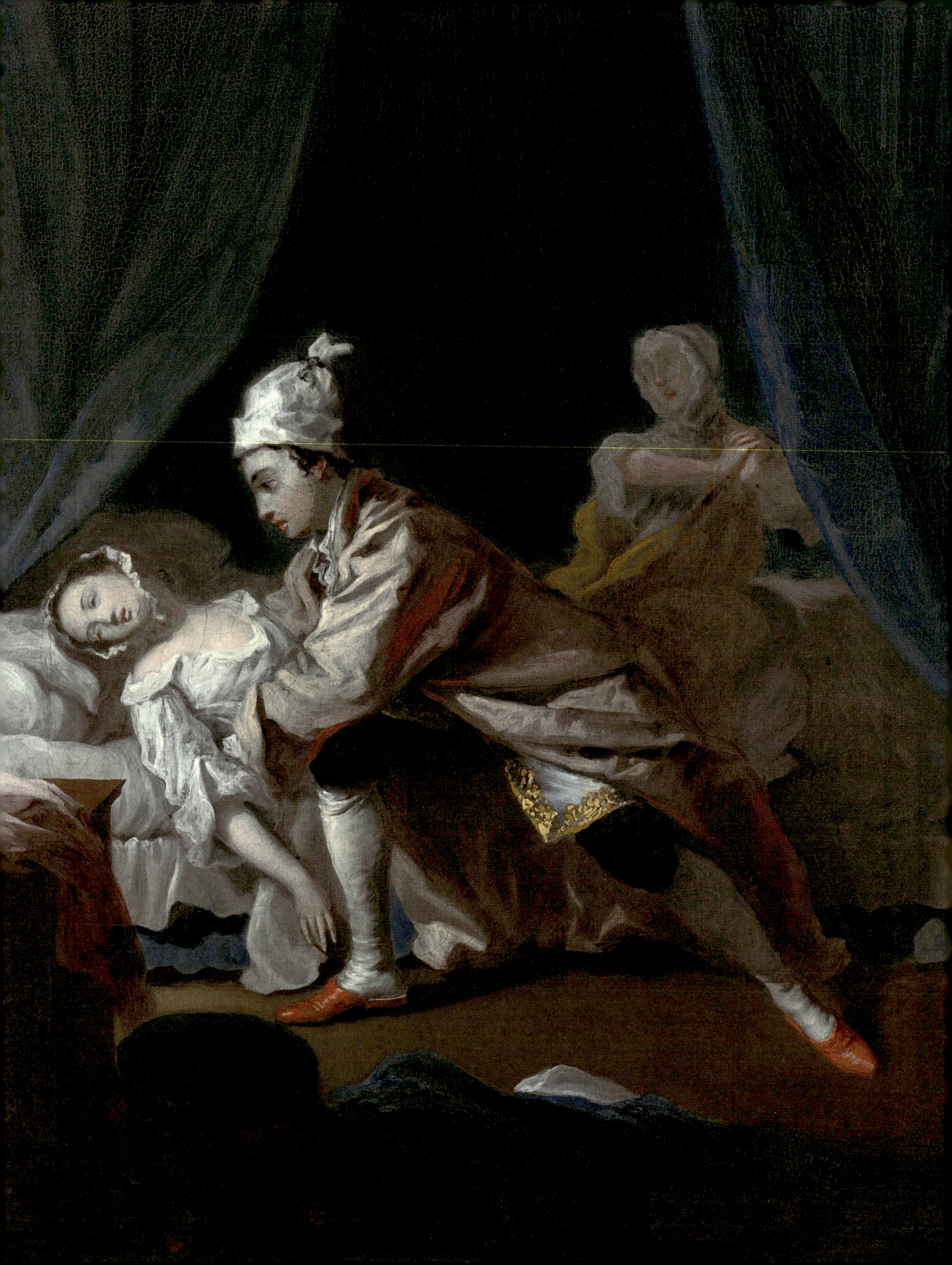

'HER WHOLE STORY'

On 16 February 1744 Joseph Highmore made an uncharacteristically bold announcement in the popular London newspaper the *General Evening Post*:

> Mr. HIGHMORE *proposes to publish by* SUBSCRIPTION, TWELVE PRINTS, by the best French Engravers, after his own PAINTINGS, representing the most remarkable *Adventures* of PAMELA: In which he has endeavoured to comprehend her whole Story; as well as to preserve a Connection between the several Pictures, which follow each other as Parts successive, and dependent, so as to compleat the Subject.[1]

Readers would have instantly identified the 'Pamela' concerned as the heroine of the novel *Pamela: or, Virtue Rewarded* by Samuel Richardson published four years earlier.[2] Rather than simply illustrating the novel, Highmore's twelve images are promoted as 'representing' a selection of events or adventures that not only focus on the most remarkable or noteworthy incidents within the novel but seek collectively to comprehend, or interpret, 'her whole Story'. The advertisement goes on to state: 'Ten of the Pictures being already finish'd, and may now be seen at Mr. *Highmore*'s House, the Two Lions in Lincoln's-Inn Fields, where Subscriptions are taken in'.[3] By 13 March 1745, Highmore could announce in the *Daily Advertiser* that 'all the twelve Pictures have been some Time finish'd, and ten of the Plates are now engrav'd'. Similar advertisements were placed in the same journal, as well as the *General Evening Post* and the *General Advertiser*, throughout March and April – the last declaring that subscription for the engravings 'will be closed this Day, the 1st May; after which they will not be sold under Two Guineas and a Half'.[4] The engravings were finally published on 1 July 1745.

This sequence of advertisements was the artist's first and last concerted use of the London press as a means of promotion, a fact that, in itself, reveals the highly speculative nature of the project. William Hogarth's 'A Harlot's Progress' of 1731 (engravings April 1732) and 'A Rake's Progress' of 1734 (engravings June 1735) were obvious prototypes, although Highmore had waited almost ten years before attempting any scheme nearing Hogarth's famous 'progresses' in scale and commercial ambition. In fact, at exactly the same time as Highmore was developing his 'Pamela' series, Hogarth was working on the paintings and overseeing the production of the engravings for his 'Marriage A-la-Mode'. Hogarth's newspaper announcement of 2 April 1743, declaring that his new series would be 'engrav'd by the very best Masters in Paris',[5] has echoes in Highmore's own announcement regarding 'the best French engravers' almost a year later.

Highmore's interest in the Hogarth model extended far beyond the use of French engravers and a multi-image format. Nor was Highmore interested in aping precisely his fellow artist's *modus operandi*. After all, the starting point for Highmore's images was a published novel, not his own imagination. Yet to the art-buying public and even to Highmore's artist peers the 'Pamela' project was similar enough to Hogarth's multi-print 'Modern Moral Subjects' for its success – or failure – to be viewed in direct comparison to these extremely popular and commercially lucrative predecessors.[6]

However, any financial risk on Highmore's part had been significantly reduced by his choice of subject. By 1743 Pamela's story was an international bestseller and a cultural and social phenomenon.[7] Highmore's project had every potential of delivering a sizable financial return, with corresponding public and artistic fame.

Highmore was not the first, or indeed the last, independently to harness Richardson's extraordinary success to his own ends. But analysis of the twelve 'adventures' the artist chose, coupled with the particular models – including examples by Hogarth – that he adapted, will reveal a very precise and distinctive approach to Pamela's history. On a basic level, the novelty of this approach would make the ownership of the engravings more appealing. On another, it might indicate the deliberate employment of this famous novel as a vehicle for a hard-hitting personal critique of modern-day society.

'TO COMPLEAT THE SUBJECT'

Richardson had always intended his novel to be a form of guide or conduct book for the young, as the early advertisements for *Pamela* in 1740 make clear:

> Pamela: Or, Virtue Rewarded .... Now first publish'd in order to cultivate the Principles of Virtue and Religion on the Minds of the Youth of both Sexes. A Narrative which has its Foundation in Truth and Nature; and at the same Time that it agreeably entertains, by a Variety of curious and affecting Incidents, is entirely divested of all those Images, which, in too many Pieces calculated for Amusement only, tend to inflame the Minds they should instruct.[8]

The novel, in the opinion of the author, provided examples of correct behaviour, guidance made more entertaining by 'a Variety of curious and affecting Incidents' – which hints that the story is constructed from a sequence of scenes that serve as moral and religious, meaning Christian, exemplars. These incidents might in turn offer a clear indication, to an artist for example, of what would be worthy of visual representation. Through the stated intention not to 'inflame the Minds' of its impressionable young readers, the advertisement intimates that the central concern is how young unmarried males and females should conduct themselves in interactions of a potentially amorous or, more bluntly, sexual nature.

The particular social setting in which Richardson chooses to broach these tensions suggests a much broader, even radical agenda. The story follows the adolescent servant girl Pamela Andrews, who is possessed of strong virtues and religious principles and who, prior to the beginning of the novel, has been working as the maid to the dowager of an aristocratic country estate. Pamela's mistress, her patron and protector, has recently died. This allows the son and heir, 'Mr. B', to give full vent to his desire for Pamela through a series of physical assaults, including abduction and attempted rape and systematic mental bullying and intimidation. Over the original two volumes, Pamela – who, crucially, is attracted to Mr B. and believes in his inherent goodness despite his behaviour – maintains and defends her chastity and principles against this relentless onslaught. Her torment is such that she briefly contemplates suicide as the only means of liberation. Finally, the example of her physical and moral virtue reforms her persecutor and they are married. Richardson immediately extended his original novel by another two volumes, entitled *Pamela in her Exalted Condition*, within which he sets out the model union of mutual respect and respectability that Mr and Mrs B. have established after their marriage – a union that sees Pamela's willing acceptance of her husband's illegitimate daughter Miss Goodwin and her own acceptance, in turn, as an admired and valued member of Mr B.'s family.

In response to this narrative, Highmore's sequence opens (fig. 34) with Mr B. entering his mother's dressing room, which Pamela has habitually used with the blessing of her late mistress. Mr B. has interrupted Pamela writing a letter to her parents, in which she informs them of his inheritance of the estate and his apparent kindness towards her. As a hint of what is to come, Mr B. is shown invading her privacy by demanding to see the letter. In Scene 2 (fig. 35) Mr B.'s real intentions towards Pamela become more than evident. He verbally and physically assaults her in the summerhouse, where she has been quietly engaged in needlework. Another servant, Mrs Jervis, who can be seen through the window, has only recently left the building in which the assault takes place. The third scene (fig. 36) portrays the moment after Mr B. has molested Pamela in the bedroom that she shares with Mrs Jervis. In Highmore's composition, Pamela has fainted in Mr B.'s arms as Mrs Jervis cries out in distress. After this traumatic encounter, Pamela prepares to return to her parents, as seen in the fourth image (fig. 37). She is pictured explaining to Mrs Jervis that she has separated her possessions into three bundles, intending to leave behind the first and second, which contain the clothes and gifts that her late mistress and Mr B. have given her. Unfortunately Mr B. is hiding in the closet and has overheard Pamela's plan.

In the fifth scene (fig. 38), ignorant of Mr B.'s scheme to abduct her, Pamela is seated in his family carriage and her fellow servants have gathered to bid her a fond farewell. Mr B. can be seen lurking at a first-floor window. Having been taken to another of Mr B.'s country estates, Pamela in the sixth scene (fig. 39) finds herself in a walled garden, enlisting the sympathetic local curate, Mr Williams, to act as the go-between for a covert exchange of letters to assist her escape. She gestures towards two tiles under which the letters will be hidden, while the grotesque housekeeper, Mrs Jewkes, is temporarily distracted from her role as Pamela's gaoler. Scene 7 (fig. 40) depicts the preamble to the most aggressive attempted rape. Mr B. has disguised himself as a drunken female servant and observes Pamela undressing. Mrs Jewkes, who is party to Mr B.'s plan, is awaiting Pamela in the bed. This attempted rape scene is the crux of the story. Pamela's extreme reaction to the combined assault of Mr B. and his accomplice Mrs Jewkes is such that Mr B. finally acknowledges the genuine nature of Pamela's defence of her chastity and is converted away from his libertine ways. This outcome is established in the next scene (fig. 41), in which Pamela appears as Mr B.'s wife-to-be in an aristocratic social gathering. The occasion is interrupted by the dignified presence of Pamela's anxious father. Mr B. looks on as daughter and father are tenderly reunited, after which Pamela sets about reassuring her parent of Mr B.'s transformation and his now honourable interest in her. She requests her father's blessing on their intended marriage. In the following scene (fig. 42) the couple are married in Mr B.'s private chapel. In Scene 10 (fig. 43), Pamela is being assaulted and insulted by Mr B.'s sister, Lady Davers, who is ignorant of Pamela's new marital status. Lady Davers believes her to be the willing recipient of Mr B.'s sexual advances and a presumptuous social climber. By the following scene (fig. 44) Lady Davers has admitted Pamela's virtuous character, while Pamela is shown earnestly charming another family member, Mr B.'s pompous uncle Sir Jacob Swinford, who has stubbornly refused to meet his nephew's 'lowborn' wife. Finally, in the twelfth scene (fig. 45), Pamela is seated among her female servants and her children, including Mr B's illegitimate daughter, telling stories that captivate and delight her audience.

Although the display of the twelve paintings was a key element of Highmore's marketing strategy, it was through the engravings by the London-based Frenchmen Antoine Benoist (1721–1770) and Louis Truchy (1721?–1764), rather than the paintings, that Highmore's personal response to Richardson's novel would be delivered to the broader art-buying public and, fundamentally, income would be generated. Each print was accompanied by a short text in English and French offering a brief explanation of the moment represented. These allow for a more precise interpretation of the artist's intentions and his choice

OVERLEAF 34–45 Louis Truchy (Plates 1, 2, 7, 8, 9, 10 and 11) and Antoine Benoist (Plates 3, 4, 5, 6 and 12) after Joseph Highmore, 'Pamela', 1745, 12 plates, each etching with stipple engraving; Plate 1, 296 x 375 mm, The British Museum, London; Plates 2 and 3, 383 x 510 mm; Plate 4, 391 x 510 mm; Plate 5, 397 x 502 mm; Plates 6, 7 and 8, 374 x 476 mm; Plates 9, 10 and 11, 390 x 540 mm; Plate 12, 393 x 541 mm, all (Plates 2–12) Yale Center for British Art, Yale Art Gallery Collection, Gift of the Library Associates

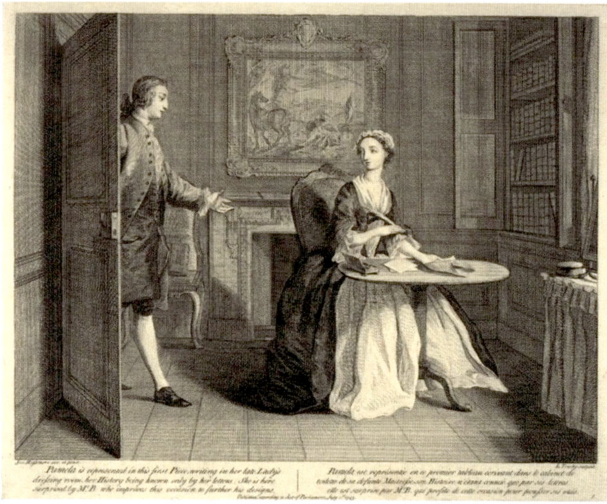

34 'Pamela', Plate 1: *Pamela writing in her late Lady's dressing room*

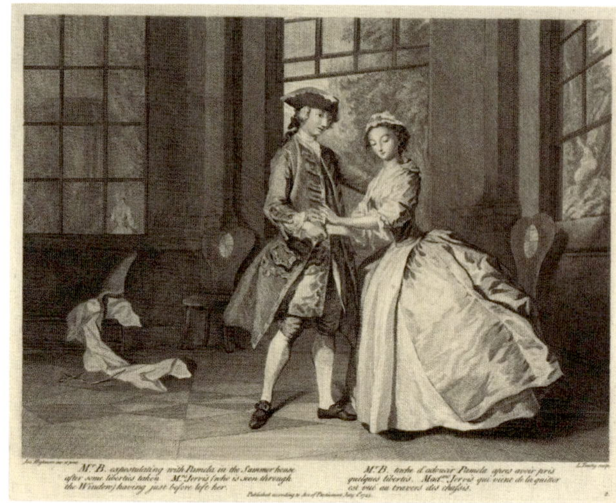

35 'Pamela', Plate 2: *Mr. B. expostulating with Pamela in the Summer house*

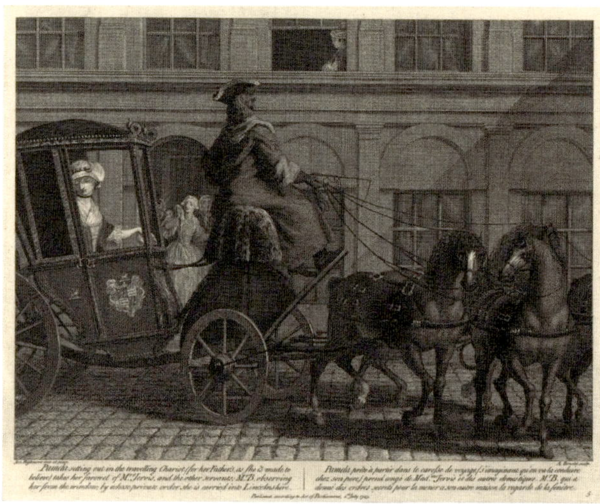

38 'Pamela', Plate 5: *Pamela setting out in the travelling Chariot*

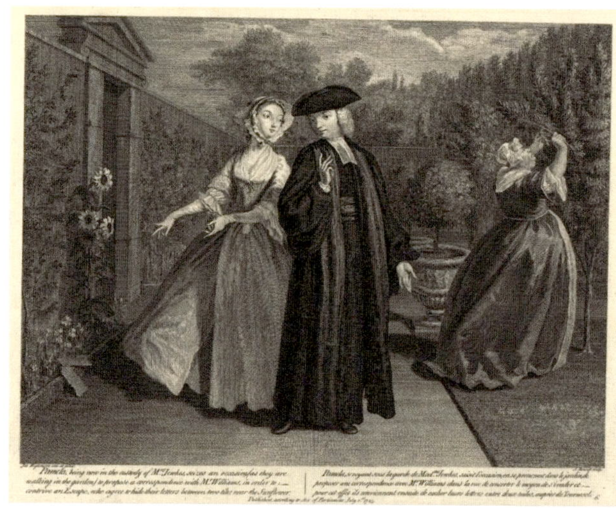

39 'Pamela', Plate 6: *Pamela ... seizes an occasion ... to propose a correspondence with Mr. Williams*

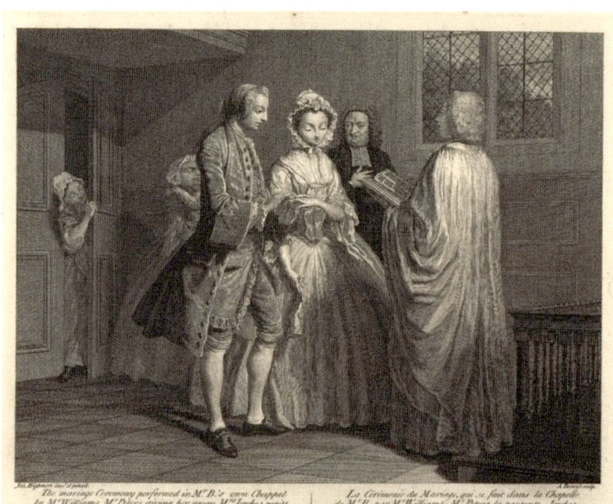

42 'Pamela', Plate 9: *The mariage Ceremony*

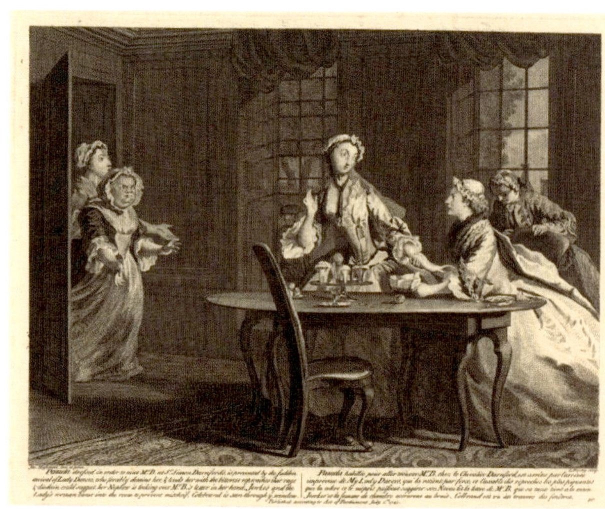

43 'Pamela', Plate 10: *Pamela dressed in order to meet Mr. B. at Sir Simon Darnford's*

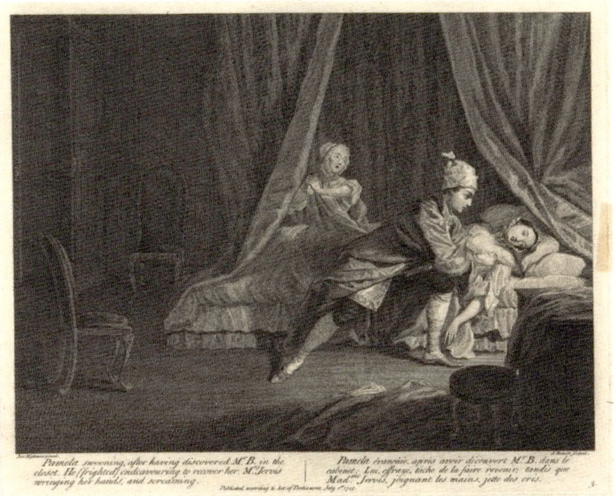

36 'Pamela', Plate 3: *Pamela swooning after having discovered Mr. B.*

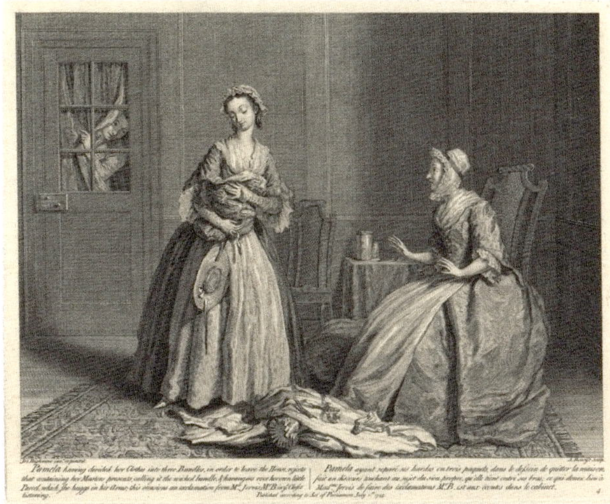

37 'Pamela', Plate 4: *Pamela having divided her Clothes into three Bundles*

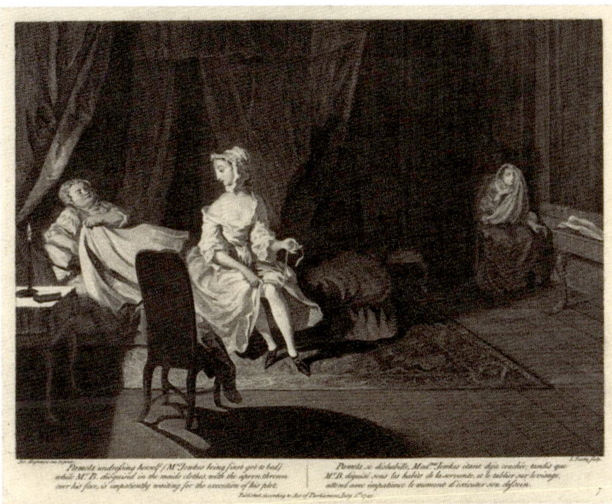

40 'Pamela', Plate 7: *Pamela undressing herself*

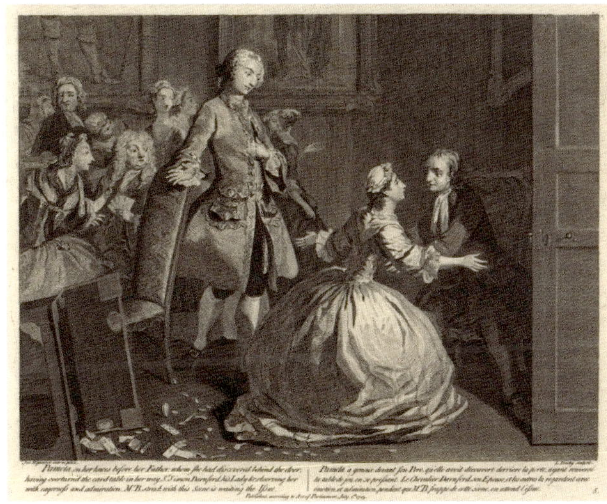

41 'Pamela', Plate 8: *Pamela on her knees before her Father*

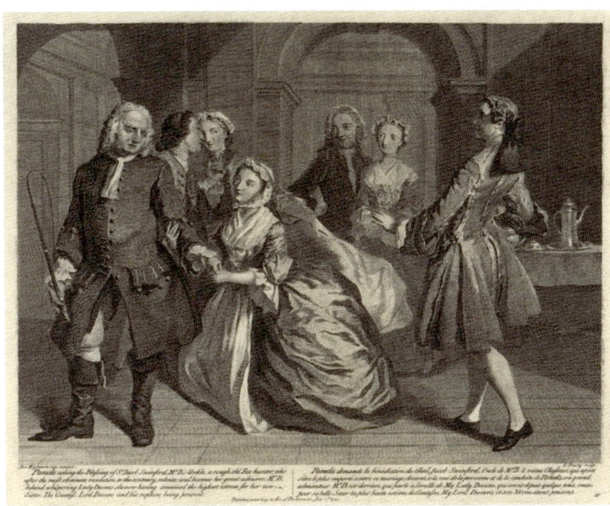

44 'Pamela', Plate 11: *Pamela asking the Blessing of Sr Jacob Swinford*

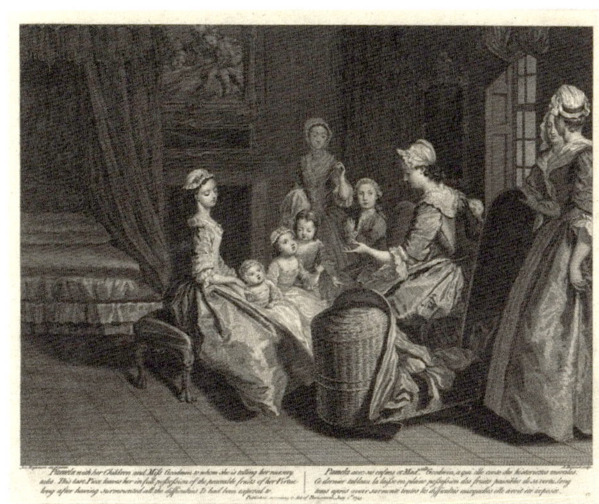

45 'Pamela', Plate 12: *Pamela with her Children and Miss Goodwin*

of narrative emphasis. However, we also know from Highmore's original advertisement of 16 February 1744 that he aimed to represent what were, in his opinion, Pamela's 'most remarkable *adventures*', which, in the event, meant the exclusion of important early scenes from the novel, including her contemplation of suicide. Despite this inevitable narrowing of focus, Highmore claims in the same advertisement to have 'endeavoured to comprehend her whole Story, as well as to preserve a Connexion between the several Pictures; which will follow each other as Parts successive, and dependent, so as to compleat the Subject'.[9]

Richardson had presented Pamela's history in the guise of original letters that were anonymously edited for publication. Here Highmore promotes himself as a fellow editor or narrator of Pamela's story, while his choice of wording suggests that the connection and dependency between these selected scenes are of his, rather than Richardson's, devising. At the very least the advertisement confirms that the intended purpose and effect of Highmore's images were not simply those of illustration. This is made clearer still by a later statement in the same advertisement, that the connection between the images 'is more distinctly illustrated in a printed Sheet given to the Subscribers, wherein all the Twelve Pictures are described, and their respective Connexions shewn'.[10] As yet, no example of this printed sheet has come to light, but its existence proves that Highmore was determined that his version of *Pamela* should be clearly understood. He had not been commissioned by Richardson to produce these images and therefore his choice of narrative and any further layers of meaning, suggested by the 'connexions', were made independently of the author.

'THE MOST REMARKABLE ADVENTURES'

Highmore's series was just one contribution to an extraordinary body of images and texts that sprang from Richardson's novel. The novel's phenomenal success immediately generated a vast array of theatrical productions, spin-offs, sequels and spoofs that either, for commercial gain, tapped into the popularity of the novel or attacked it.[11] Richardson's revisions to the original text and his production of two further volumes, covering Pamela's marriage and motherhood, suggest that he was extremely concerned about the effects of early 'anti-Pamelist' ridicule. These writers, most famously – and devastatingly – Henry Fielding in his *An Apology for the Life of Mrs Shamela Andrews* (published 1741), exploited the ambiguities and titillations of the original text to satirize and eroticize the young servant girl.[12] In *Shamela*, Richardson's heroine has been transformed into a conniving, social-climbing harlot, who conducts an affair with Parson Williams while she manoeuvres the gormless 'Mr. Booby' into marriage.

Highmore may have been aware that Richardson had approached William Hogarth to produce two frontispieces for the second edition of *Pamela* (1741). Sadly neither design was published and the originals have never been traced.[13] It has been suggested that Richardson rejected Hogarth's interpretation of Pamela because it had veered towards a satirical Shamela spin.[14] This is a well-worn oversimplification of Hogarth's artistic and intellectual drive, and one which ignores his declared ambitions in 'elevated' art forms including history painting. In any case, Richardson's next commission proved more ambitious and successful. Twenty-nine illustrations of the novel by Francis Hayman (1708–1776) and Hubert Gravelot were published in the sixth edition, of 1742, and are the most significant visual precedent for Highmore's series.[15] Two of Hayman's designs were used for paintings decorating supper boxes at Vauxhall Pleasure Gardens (unveiled c.1742).[16] As a result, these author-commissioned illustrations existed in formats within both private and public spaces – an indication of the versatility as well as popularity of Richardson's creation. Crucially, as part of the pro-Pamela counterattack, they offered Highmore a dignified graphic as well as narrative model. It is certain that the author maintained a strict control over his artists.[17] Hayman and Gravelot were also required to give even weight to all four volumes. However, in sharp contrast to Highmore, there is a complete absence within their designs of any sexually charged scenes or imagery, although the moment when Pamela contemplates suicide – which many readers would have considered equally distressing – is included. This establishes an immediate separation from Highmore's later selection, which, when balanced with the four volumes of Richardson's text, signals a preference for specific narrative threads.

To be precise, the two original volumes were Highmore's focus, with seven images deriving from the first volume and three from the second. In contrast the third and fourth volumes are allotted only one image each. Highmore has not so much edited as filleted Richardson's novel. As a result, the imagery is significantly weighted towards Pamela's early trials and the defence of her virtue, rather than lingering over her elevation to the social elite. Indeed, in devoting over half of his images to the events leading up to and including the most aggressive attempted rape, Highmore reveals a particular interest in the period when Pamela's physical and mental suffering, in defence of her virtue, is at its most extreme and violent. Pertinent to this emphasis is Highmore's later published statement: '[V]irtue that exposes not a man to suffering deserves little praise or reward. Virtue ought never to shrink, or give way in the least, nor does, without forfeiting so much of its value.'[18] This last sentiment may suggest why Highmore excluded any reference to Pamela escaping her torment through suicide.

Despite the glaring differences between the two sequences, there are seven scenes or events that broadly correspond across the two projects – Mr B. interrupting Pamela writing, the first image in both sequences; Pamela preparing to leave; the arrival of her father; the marriage; Lady Davers abusing Pamela; Pamela and Sir Jacob Swinford; and Pamela with her children (the last scene in both). Comparison between a selection of the Hayman-Gravelot designs and Highmore's printed scenes will begin to clarify the latter's specific approach to Pamela's history.

One of Hayman's illustrations (fig. 46), located opposite page 123 of the first volume of this sixth edition, corresponds with the fourth scene of Highmore's 'Pamela'. It shows Pamela preparing to leave Mr B.'s house and describing the contents of the three bundles to Mrs Jervis. The first contains the items, including clothing, that 'my good Lady gave me'; the second is described as the 'wicked' bundle, containing the 'gifts', or rather bribes, that Mr B. has given Pamela as 'the Price of my Shame'.[19] The third contains the items she plans to take home with her. Though not obvious from the illustration itself, its placing within the text suggests that the bundle lying on the floor, towards which Pamela is gesturing in Hayman's design, is the third bundle. Hayman places Mr B. behind the two women, drawing back a tall curtain that barely conceals his presence.

In the fourth scene of Highmore's 'Pamela' (fig. 47), the artist explicitly chooses to represent the moment where Pamela is holding the third or 'modest' bundle containing her own clothes, as his text makes clear.[20] In the novel, Pamela declares, 'come to my Arms, my dear *third* Parcel, the Companion of my Poverty, and the Witness of my Honesty'.[21] Highmore's text states that she 'harangues' over this bundle, a reminder of her impassioned speech supporting honourable poverty, dignity and integrity over dishonour in exchange for material wealth. This action, as described by Highmore's text, 'occasions an exclamation from Mrs. Jervis', a signal of her admiration for Pamela's moral superiority. In sympathy with this, Highmore depicts Pamela standing or 'upright', bathed in a dazzling light that contrasts with the darkness dominating the right half of the image. This last detail directly responds to Richardson's stated intention for his novel, as set out in the preface, '*to set* VIRTUE *in its own amiable Light, to make it look* Lovely'.[22]

As a result of this illumination, Pamela's figure casts a long shadow, which stretches across the floor and then upwards to the door, behind which Mr B. is hiding, as if it has become a giant accusatory finger. In contrast to the Hayman-Gravelot version, Mr B.'s crouched, almost comic posture in the small closet at the back of the room, trapped as he is behind the closed door and window bars, suggests that he is not only imprisoned by his actions and desires, but barred or blocked – by circumstances or wilful self-delusion – from Pamela's

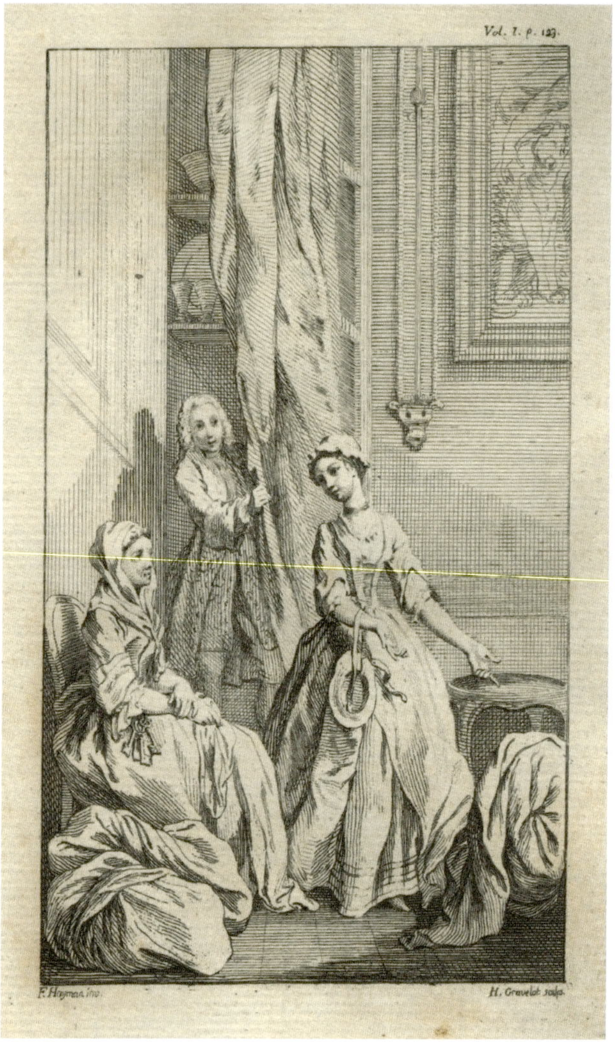

46 Hubert Gravelot after Francis Hayman, Illustration to Samuel Richardson's *Pamela: or, Virtue Rewarded*, 1742, 6th edition, vol. 1, page 123, etching, 128 x 74 mm, The William Ready Division of Archives and Research Collections, McMaster University Library

virtuous example and 'light'. Highmore has therefore set out, to use Richardson's own metaphor, '*to paint* VICE *in its proper Colours, to make it* deservedly Odious'.[23] This image sets up a marked contrast between the dignified and honourable actions of Mr B.'s servants, which have been accordingly foregrounded, in opposition to his own undignified, inelegant and ultimately un-gentlemanly behaviour, which has been symbolically set back, enclosed and therefore disparagingly belittled.

The illustration in the second volume opposite page 89 (fig. 48) corresponds with the eighth scene of Highmore's 'Pamela' series. Gravelot's setting is an elegant drawing room where Pamela's father has risen from his seat, behind the door, to embrace his daughter, who stands before him. Pamela has turned over a card table in her distracted haste to reach her father, while the assembled party have all risen to witness the reunion. Highmore has presented a different moment, when Pamela kneels before her seated father (figs. 49 and 50). The engraving subtext reads, 'Pamela on her knees before her Father; whom she had discovered behind the door: having overturn'd the card-table in her way'. Rather than being pushed back into the composition, the toppled card table – here symbolic perhaps of aristocratic idleness and self-indulgence – is shown prominently in the left foreground, the chips and cards dotting the floor towards the figure of Pamela to the right. The text therefore emphasizes that Pamela has dropped from the 'elevated' standing position of Mr B. to join her father: in truth, she has reduced herself or 'sunk', as she herself describes it, so as to be just below him in a posture of supplication and deference. To achieve this she has, without hesitation, cast aside the card table that was blocking her way.

Pamela and her father, in their physically lowered poses, remain isolated in one half of the room, while the assembled aristocrats, some standing, some seated still holding their cards, are crammed into the other. Despite Highmore's accompanying text stating that 'S^{r}. Simon Darnford, his Lady &c observing her with eagerness and admiration', in reality none of them, as depicted here, seem truly capable of comprehending, or even actively responding to, the display of genuine feeling and filial-paternal love and respect occurring in their midst. As if to visualize this challenge to their insipid aristocratic equilibrium, the full-length ancestral paintings hanging behind them (of Highmore's devising) are strategically 'cut off' at the knees. Highmore's message seems to be that Pamela may be joining the ranks of the landed classes, indeed may be admired by them, as Richardson makes clear, but she will always remain separated from

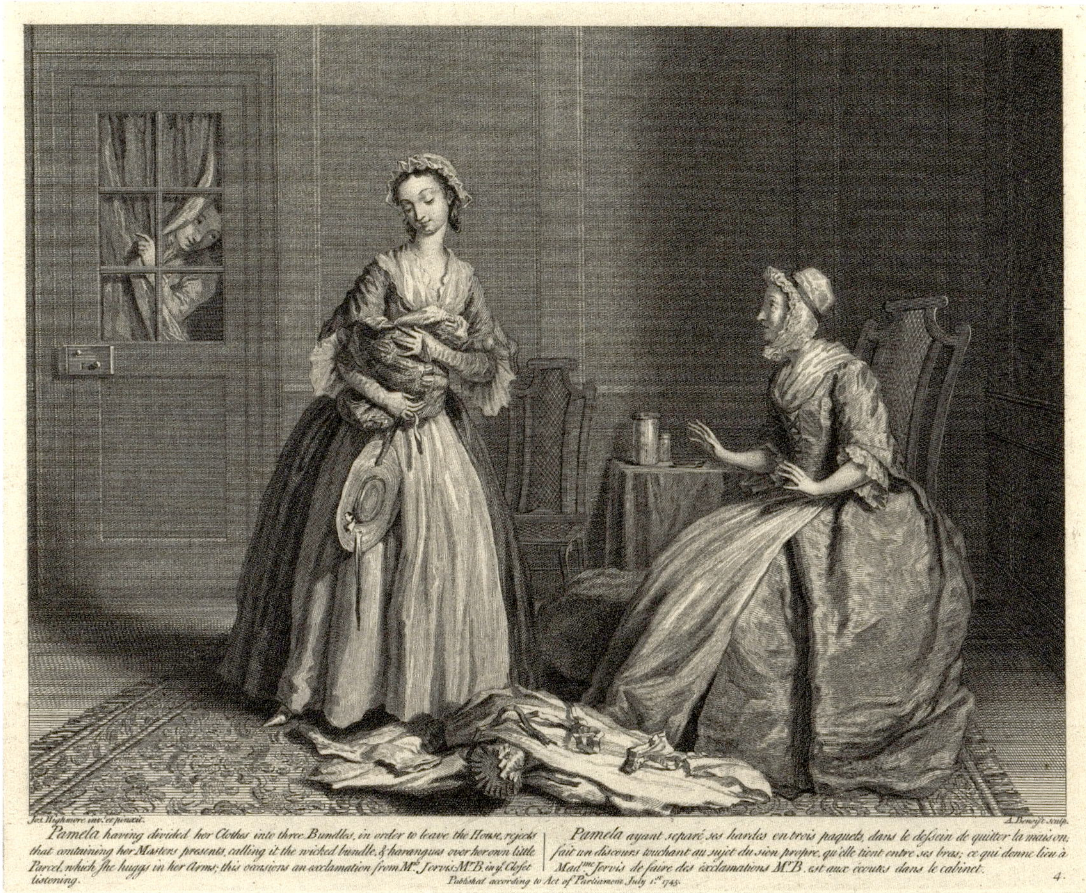
Jos. Highmore inv. et pinxit.
A. Benoist sculp.
Pamela having divided her Clothes into three Bundles, in order to leave the House, rejects that containing her Masters presents, calling it the wicked bundle, & harangues over her own little Parcel, which she huggs in her Arms; this occasions an exclamation from Mrs. Jervis: Mr. B. in ye Closet listening.
Pamela ayant separé ses hardes en trois paquets, dans le dessein de quitter la maison, fait un discours touchant au sujet du sien propre, qu'elle tient entre ses bras; ce qui donne lieu à Madme. Jervis de faire des éxclamations Mr. B. est aux écoutes dans le cabinet.
Publishd according to Act of Parliament July 1st 1745.
4.

47 'Pamela', Plate 4: *Pamela having divided her Clothes into three Bundles*

this group through her natural humility and honesty of feeling. However, for the first time Highmore allows Mr B. to have the awareness and refinement of feeling to be 'struck with this Scene'.[24] Highmore represents him with his hand tucked into his coat, a recognizably genteel stance, as a visible signal of his return to the elevated and refined attitudes, as well as the social status, of an ideal gentleman.

The final scene in both sets comes from the extended novel's fourth volume. The two images show Pamela seated among her children and female servants, telling morally uplifting stories. In Gravelot's design (fig. 51) the scene is of balance and happiness revolving around the person and personality of Pamela herself. Highmore appears to have rotated Gravelot's composition through 180° (figs. 52 and 53). In the engraving, Pamela now sits to the right with her back to us, the maids standing behind her chair are now located to the right and pulled forward, and the children sit in a row before Pamela, facing forward. This transforms the composition and its meaning. In Highmore's version, Miss Goodwin, Mr B.'s illegitimate daughter, is given a much greater presence: her face tilts elegantly forward and her left hand is pictured gently holding the little fingers of the infant, her half-sibling, sitting beside her. To stress her presence as an equal in this family group, Highmore names her in the accompanying text. In fact Miss Goodwin is the device that connects this scene of domestic contentment with the painting above the fireplace, of a mother figure and infants, which, in the

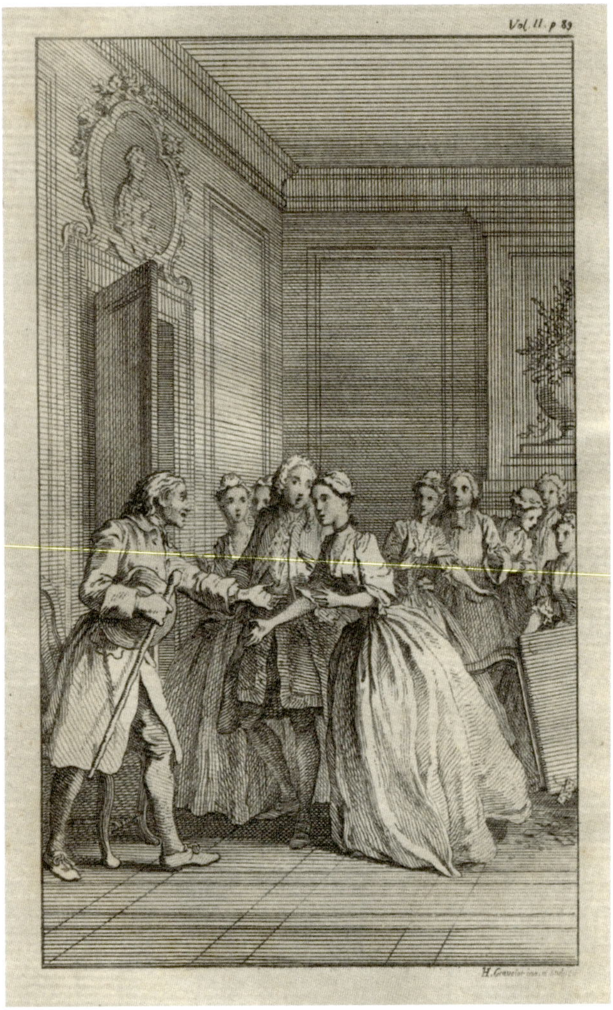

48 Hubert Gravelot, Illustration to Samuel Richardson's *Pamela: or, Virtue Rewarded*, 1742, 6th edition, vol. 2, page 89, etching, 127 x 76 mm, The William Ready Division of Archives and Research Collections, McMaster University Library

FACING
49 Joseph Highmore, 'Pamela', VIII: *Pamela on her knees before her Father*, 1743–44, oil on canvas, 63.5 x 76.2 cm, National Gallery of Victoria, Melbourne, Felton Bequest, 1921 (1116-3)

50 'Pamela', Plate 8: *Pamela on her knees before her Father*

first instance, mirrors Pamela and her offspring, but also reflects the broader theological virtue of *caritas* or love of mankind – a virtue Pamela has demonstrated in her complete acceptance of Mr B.'s illegitimate child and her general behaviour throughout the novel. This detail, again, is of Highmore's devising.

The full tester bed, in dramatic contrast to those pictured in the third and seventh scenes, is revealed to be a serene, orderly haven rather than a place of fear, disorder and defilement. Highmore's own attitude towards sexual relations (in the context of a partnership) is revealed in the following remark, published sixteen years after the death of his wife Susanna:

> As to the pleasure arising from mutual commerce of the sexes, it will certainly be acknowledged, that the highest of that kind must arise between persons entirely agreeable to each other, that is, in mind, as well as body; and where the esteem and affection are reciprocal: the most abandoned must allow this is to be wished, and that the pleasure cannot be complete otherwise.[25]

The Vigor Family (see fig. 33) is exactly contemporary with Highmore's 'Pamela' and appears to represent, precisely, this type of mature mutual attraction, respect, esteem and affection, which Highmore advocates as the foundation of a successful marriage.

Finally, the compositional rotation brings into prominence the cot and the creation of offspring, in early Georgian Britain a key, if not the key, purpose and expected outcome of marriage. It also allows for a beautifully painted and affectionately observed row of wide-eyed and pink-cheeked infants. In this sense the prominent bed acts as a visual and ideological support to the wicker cradle and the children. All represent Pamela's attainment, within marriage, of sexual, familial, domestic and maternal contentment.

Through such comparisons, a shift in emphasis between the images created under the auspices of the author and those created independently by Highmore is emerging. Richardson's novel was constructed as a sequence of 'incidents' from which moral lessons

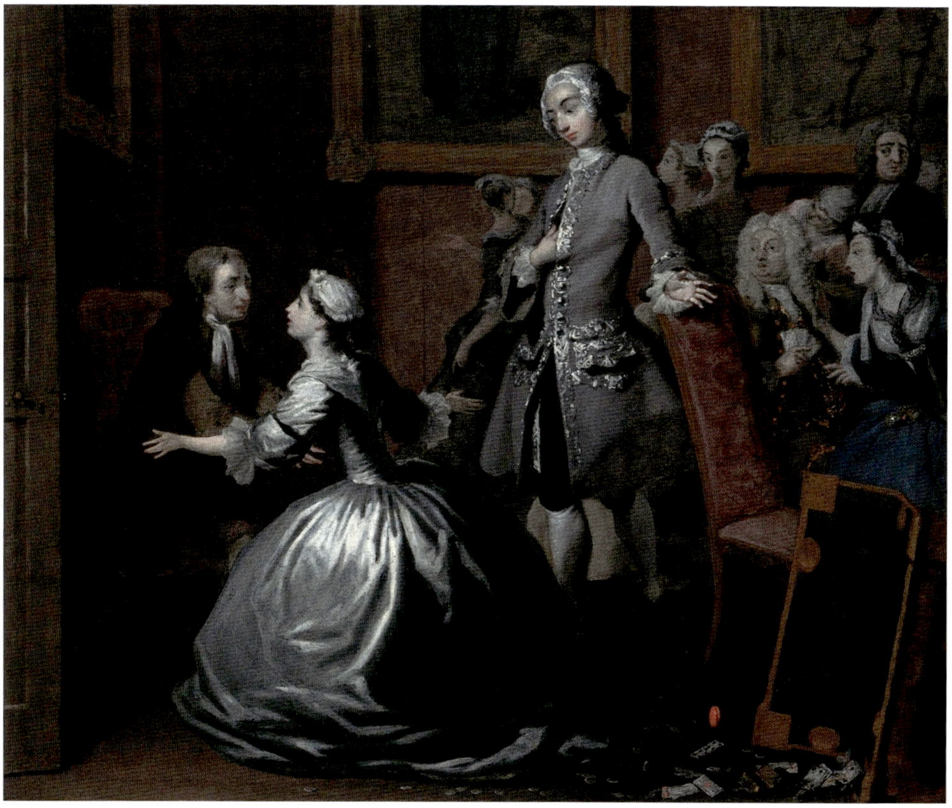

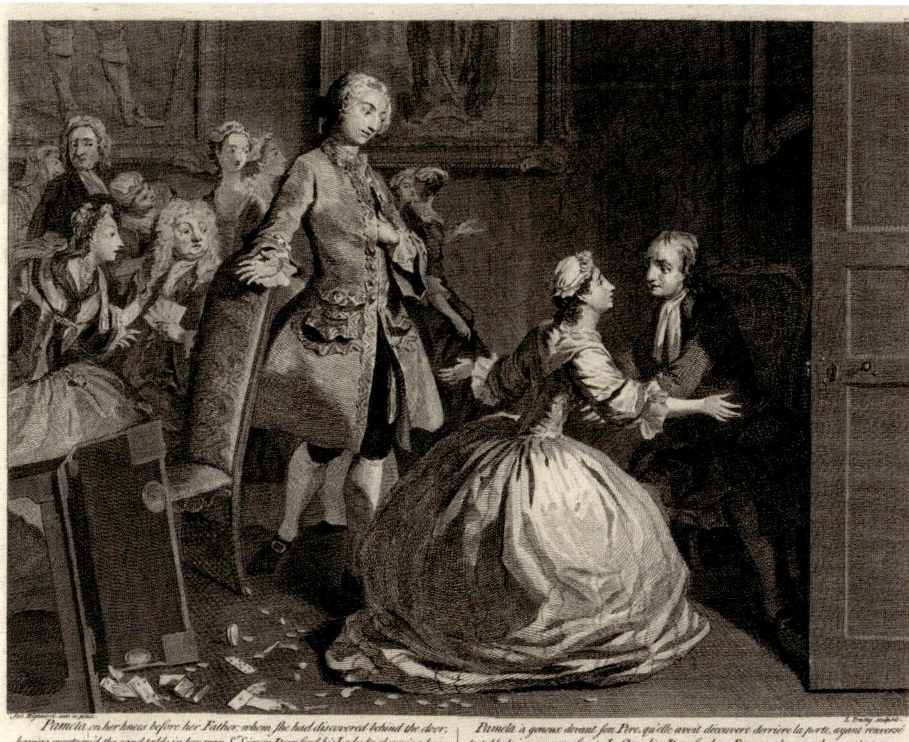

Pamela on her knees before her Father; whom she had discovered behind the door; having overturn'd the card table in her way. Sr Simon Darnford, his Lady &c. observing her with eagerness and admiration. Mr B. struck with this Scene is waiting the Issue.

Pamela à genoux devant son Pere, qu'elle avoit découvert derriere la porte, ayant renversé la table de jeu en se pressant. Le Chevalier Darnford, son Epouse, et les autres la regardent avec émotion, et admiration, pendant que Mr B. frappé de cette scene, en attend l'issue.

Published, according to Act of Parliament, July 1.st 1745.

8.

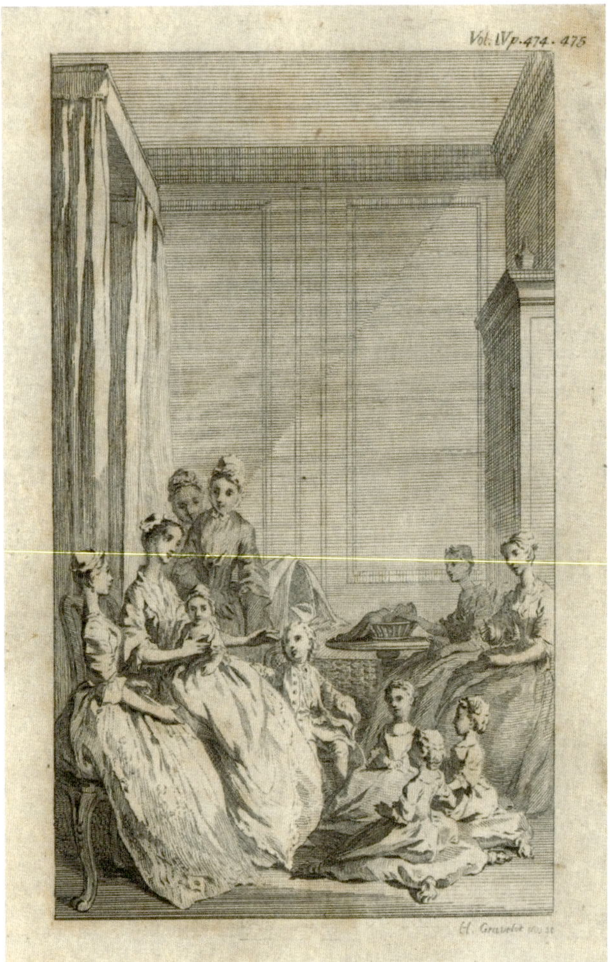

51 Hubert Gravelot, Illustration to Samuel Richardson's *Pamela: or, Virtue Rewarded,* 1742, 6th edition, vol. 4, page 474, etching, 127 x 76 mm, The William Ready Division of Archives and Research Collections, McMaster University Library

FACING
52 Joseph Highmore, 'Pamela', XII: *Pamela tells a Nursery Tale,* 1743–44, oil on canvas, 629 x 747 mm, The Fitzwilliam Museum, Cambridge

53 'Pamela', Plate 12: *Pamela with her Children and Miss Goodwin*

could be drawn. Highmore's editorial and narrative freedom as to what these key lessons might be is established, first, by his selection from the dozens of incidents offered by Richardson over the four volumes, and secondly, by his response to the images produced by Hayman and Gravelot. Highmore's twelve scenes, and the lessons contained within them, are refined through the selection of a precise moment from the episode chosen – for example, the moment when Pamela holds the third bundle, or when the father sits rather than stands – which is then honed still further by compositional choices – his decision to show Mr B. 'imprisoned' in the closet; to give prominence to the discarded card table; to include a painting of Charity. In so doing, as I will elaborate, Highmore stresses specific social concerns, which are fundamental to Richardson's overall moral aims yet are only occasionally hinted at in the Gravelot-Hayman designs.

'VIRTUE' AND 'VICE'

Further insight into Highmore's intentions can be gleaned through analysis of other relevant artistic models. As previously observed, the Benoist-Truchy engravings after Highmore would have been viewed in relation to print culture in general and, more specifically, Hogarth's 'progresses'. In fact all three of Hogarth's series would have been prominent in the public consciousness during the first half of 1745. Hogarth had advertised the publishing and sale of the second impression of the 'Harlot' in early January.[26] Soon after, on 25 January, he announced the extraordinary sale of the original paintings for the 'Rake', 'Harlot' and 'Marriage A-la-Mode', with bids being taken throughout February.[27] That the subscribers for the 'Marriage A-la-Mode' and 'Pamela' sets were not mutually exclusive is revealed by a letter from Highmore's son Anthony to Lancelot Lee dated 13 June 1745 (that is, after the publication of 'Marriage A-la-Mode' but before the 'Pamela' engravings were completed), in which Anthony states:

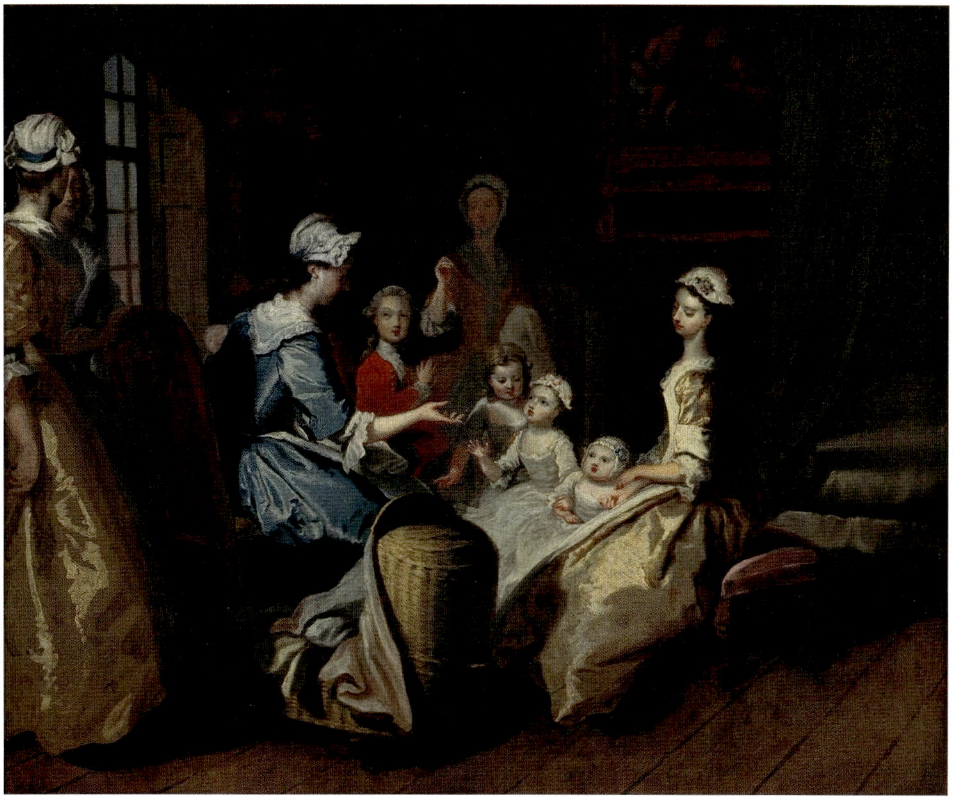

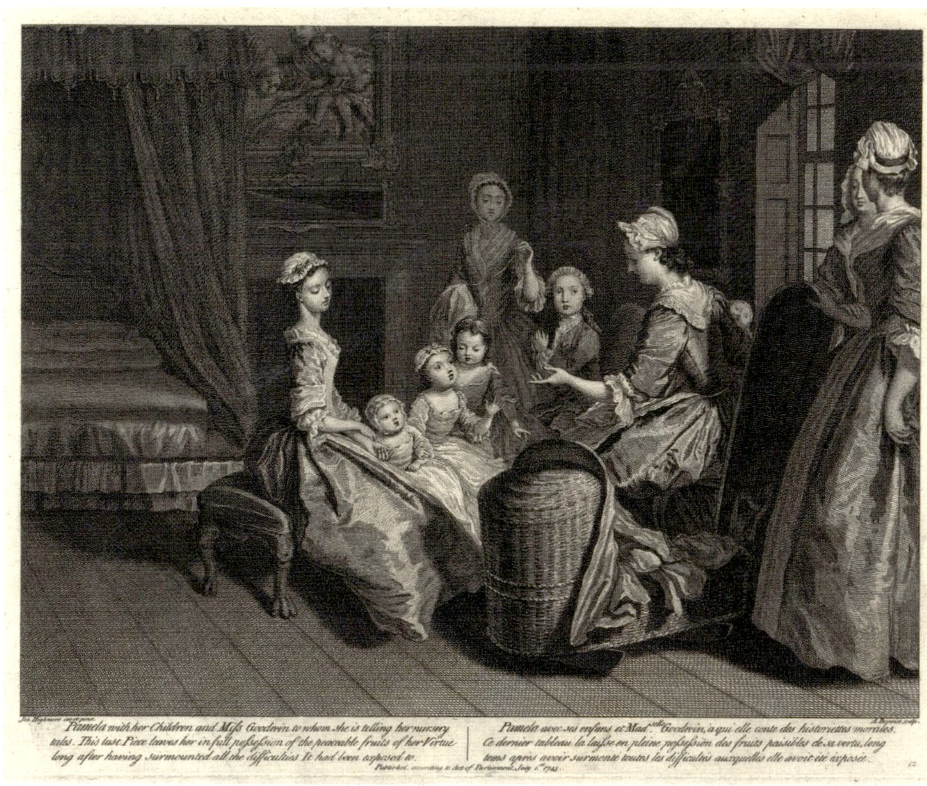
Pamela with her Children and Miss Goodwin to whom she is telling her nursery tales. This last Piece leaves her in full possession of the peaceable fruits of her Virtue long after having surmounted all the difficulties It had been exposed to.
Pamela avec ses enfans et Mad.elle Goodwin, à qui elle conte des historiettes morales. Ce dernier tableau la laisse en pleine possession des fruits paisibles de sa vertu, long tems après avoir surmonté toutes les difficultés auxquelles elle avoit été exposée.
Publish'd according to Act of Parliament, July 1st 1745.
12

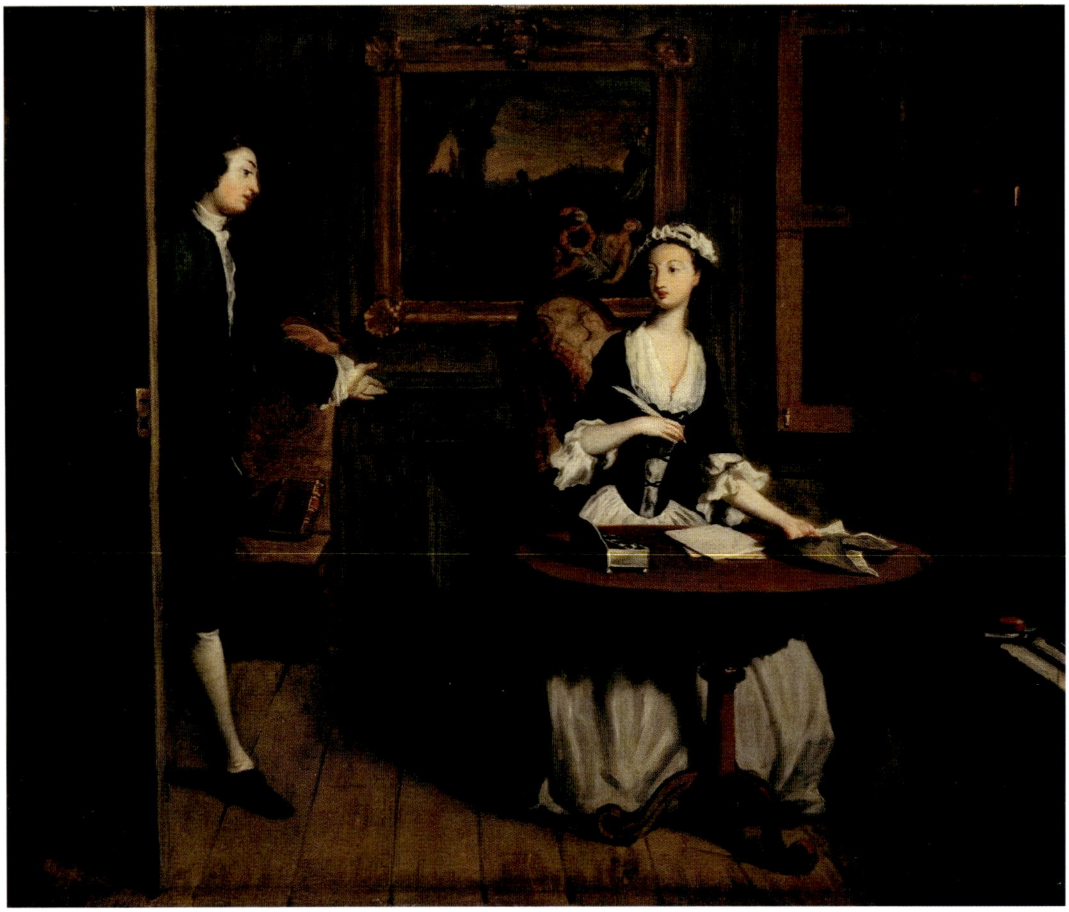

54 Joseph Highmore, 'Pamela', I: *Mr. B. finds Pamela writing*, 1743–44, oil on canvas, 65.1 x 75.9 cm, Tate

> My Prints [of Kensington and Hampton Court Palaces] are finish'd and all the subscribers have received their sets except you, but suppose you would have them with Mr. Hogarth's and my Father's. Mr. Hogarth's are deliver'd now, and if you chuse I should take them for you; please to enclose your receipt in a letter & I will take them, and also my Father's when finish'd and then do with them as you shall direct.[28]

Clearly, throughout this six-month period, Highmore and Hogarth were both vigorously promoting important commercial enterprises, a circumstance that surely generated excitement in the London art world. At the same time and as a result, Highmore's imagery of the virtuous Pamela was jostling for public attention with that of the 'Harlot', the 'Rake' and the protagonists of 'Marriage A-la-Mode', the Earl and Countess Squanderfield. Whether a coincidence or not, this would encourage direct comparison between their respective characters and histories.

In Highmore's first scene (fig. 54), the dressing room is not described by Richardson and therefore the details represented are, once again, of Highmore's creation. The open bookcase and the volume placed on the chair imply a mind open to knowledge and learning, stressing the impact of a privileged education on Pamela's character and, thereby, the progress of her history. Her manner is entirely that of a woman at ease in this world. As a result this scene, with Mr B. entering the room, could be mistaken for a portrait of

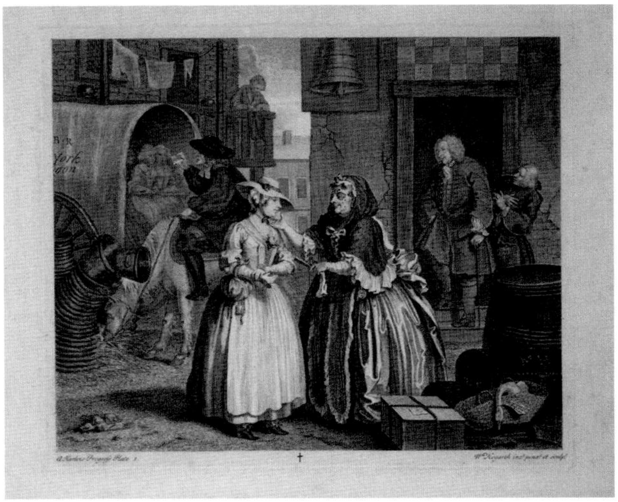

55 William Hogarth, 'A Harlot's Progress', Plate 1, 1732, etching and engraving, 318 x 383 mm, The Garrick Club, London

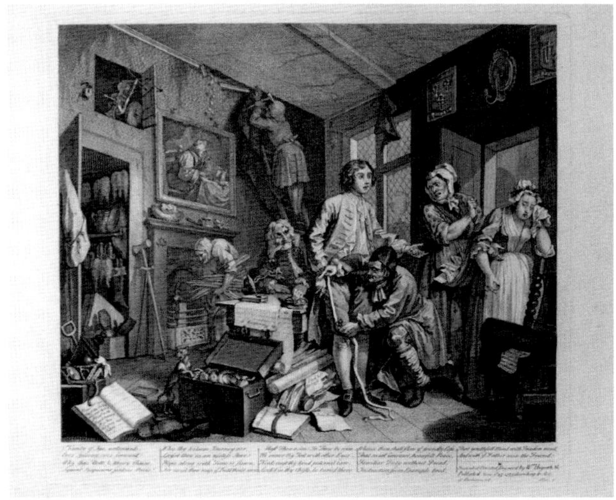

56 William Hogarth, 'A Rake's Progress', Plate 1: *The Rake taking Possession of his Estate*, 1735, etching and engraving, 350 x 404 mm, The Garrick Club, London

domestic felicity – not unlike the scenario presented in Highmore's *The Artist and his Family* (see fig. 6) – and a marriage of equals – precisely what Mr B. and Pamela achieve by the end of the novel.

Highmore's inclusion of the Christian parable of the Good Samaritan as a painting above the fireplace, however, is the key indication that this is not the case at the start of the novel and graphic sequence. The parable specifically encourages compassion towards a fellow human who is both vulnerable and in distress, and, in this sense, it refers to Pamela's present or immediate future rather than her recent past. Its significance at the beginning of Mr B. and Pamela's journey is, in part, to indicate what kind of behaviour he should adopt following his full possession of responsibility and authority. Mr B. therefore has a choice to display either charitable or uncharitable behaviour, a choice that the biblical Samaritan, Priest and Levite are also offered within their given scenario. Mr B. must also resist or override his 'baser' instincts and reveal himself to be worthy of his inherited elevated social position. An amplification of the parable Proverbs 3: 27 – 'Withhold not good from them to whom it is due, when it is in the power of thine hand to do it'[29] – might add potential meaning to Mr B.'s gesture as he enters the room – that of the open extended hand, which could mean friendship and charitable assistance but, as we are soon to discover, is merely a domineering action in demand of Pamela's letter.

In fact Mr B. chooses not only to pursue a course of uncharitable behaviour but to ape an established aristocratic male archetype, the libertine or rake, a figure at once egotistical, voracious, predatory and unchecked by religious or moral concerns.[30] Worse still, within some aristocratic circles, such behaviour, it was thought, was not only rife but condoned, as long as no woman of status was involved. Particularly vulnerable were young unmarried female servants – the scenario presented in Richardson's novel. Rape was a capital offence, whatever the social background, yet it was perceived that the social elite – as represented by the libertine – believed themselves above the law. The sensational case of Colonel Francis Charteris (c.1675–1732), nicknamed the 'Rape-Master General' – who was finally tried at the Old Bailey in 1730 for the rape of his servant Anne Bond, found guilty, sentenced to death, but pardoned (with his property later restored to him) – seemed to confirm that there was one rule for the upper classes and another for everyone else.

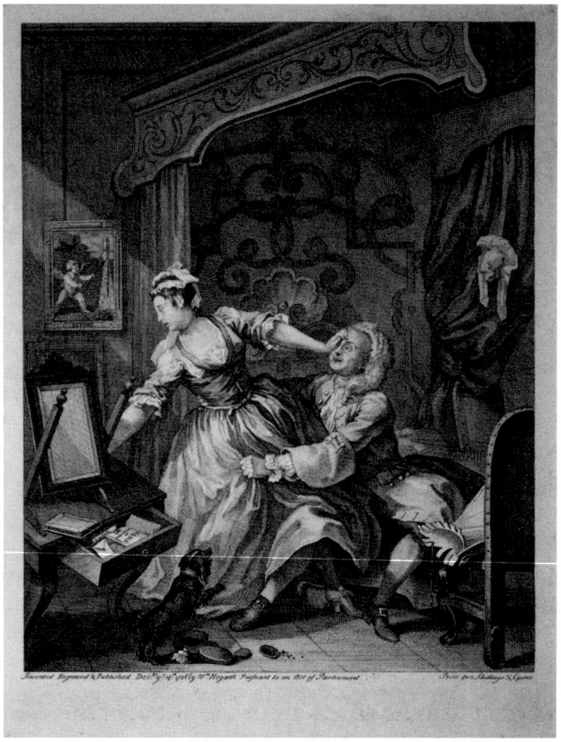

57 William Hogarth, *Before*, 1736, etching and engraving, 406 x 325 mm, The Garrick Club, London

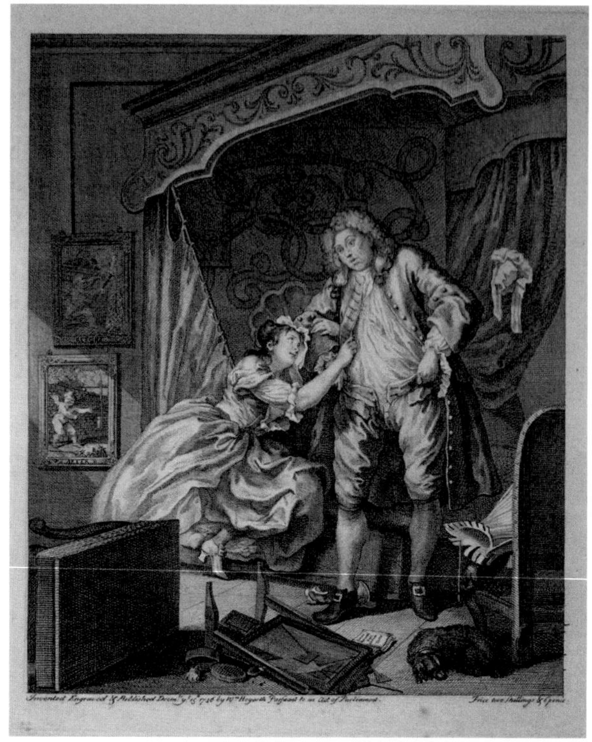

58 William Hogarth, *After*, 1736, etching and engraving, 407 x 332 mm, The Garrick Club, London

Such perceptions lie at the heart of Hogarth's progresses and in this way his 'Harlot' and 'Rake' can be viewed as contemporary antecedents to the characters of both Pamela and Mr B. The moral choices made by this couple within their respective journeys offer a virtuous alternative to Hogarth's progresses. Although in the first plate of 'A Harlot's Progress' (fig. 55) the young Moll Hackabout, an innocent girl, newly arrived from the country, is clearly preyed upon by the brothelkeeper Mother Needham (a real, rather than fictional character), with the debauched aristocrat (recognizably Charteris) awaiting his next victim at the brothel entrance, it is still the case that, at the exact moment depicted, Moll has a choice to follow or not a life of prostitution. Meanwhile, in the first scene of 'A Rake's Progress' (fig. 56), the newly wealthy Tom Rakewell has made his choice to follow the path of the dissipated libertine, and is paying off the weeping girl he has made pregnant – a scenario that is echoed in Mr B.'s earlier relationship with Sally Godfrey, Miss Goodwin's mother, and, as is made clear by his subsequent actions, a future he had intended for Pamela too.

Highmore establishes the relevance and therefore connection with Hogarth's earlier works through the choice of specific compositional signs and signals. In the first instance this is to register the recent artistic pedigree of this graphic format.[31] The selected visual associations would have been instantly recognizable to the knowing audience and therefore their presence, within this new context, would provide additional layers and meanings to Highmore's images. An exploration of two scenes will serve as examples.

Hogarth's 1736 version of *Before* and *After* (figs. 57 and 58) depicts a violent sexual assault, evident from the woman's desperate struggle and terrified expression, the crashing furniture and her assailant's grasping hands dragging her to the bed.

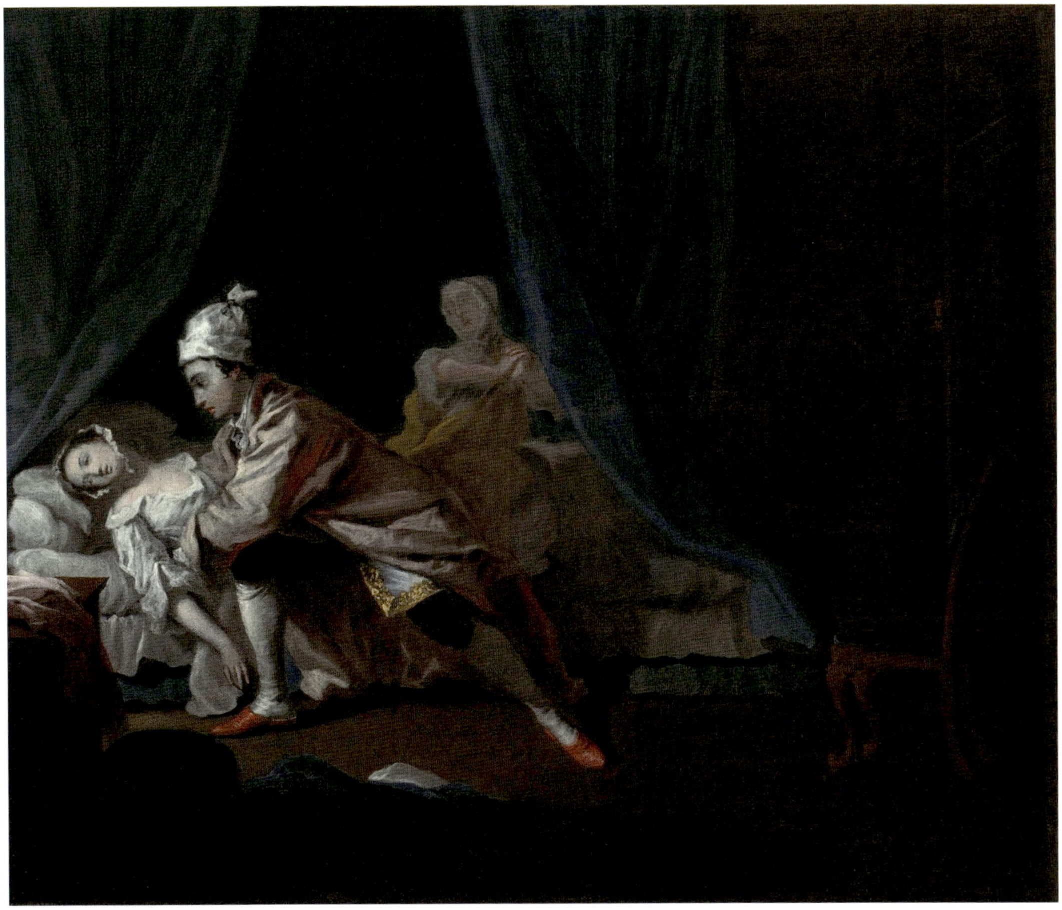

59 Joseph Highmore, 'Pamela', III: *Pamela fainting*, 1743–44, oil on canvas, 63.5 x 76.2 cm, National Gallery of Victoria, Melbourne, Felton Bequest, 1921 (1114-3)

The destruction of her virtue is revealed in the second engraving. These two images offer an explicit depiction of the reality and immediate consequence of Moll Hackabout's 'off stage' debauchment by Charteris between Scenes 1 and 2 of 'A Harlot's Progress', which sets in train her transformation from naïve girl to concubine.[32] Highmore, in his second and third 'Pamela' scenes, has pulled together the two events, the summerhouse assault and the first attempted rape (fig. 59), although they do not directly follow each other in the text. The result is the creation of a type of Before and After juxtaposition, which refers to the immediate (as seen in Hogarth's paired engravings) as well as long-term consequences (as set out in 'A Harlot's Progress') should Mr B.'s assault in either instance be successful. The rapid movement of Mr B. and Pamela from summerhouse to bedroom is most effectively charted in the prints, from left to right, rather than the paintings (see figs 35 and 36) – a hint as to the 'connections' Highmore deliberately created between his engraved images.

The association between Pamela and Moll is most self-consciously and therefore strategically made within the seventh scene of Highmore's 'Pamela'. In the third scene of 'A Harlot's Progress' (fig. 60) Hogarth calculatingly presents his viewers with the appealing image of a young, desirable and semi-clad prostitute. Moll looks out directly and provocatively, apparently

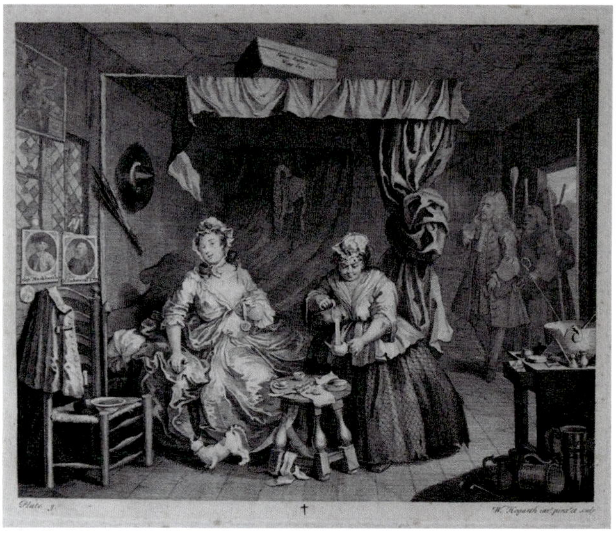

60 William Hogarth, 'A Harlot's Progress', Plate 3, 1732, etching and engraving, 318 x 383 mm, The Garrick Club, London

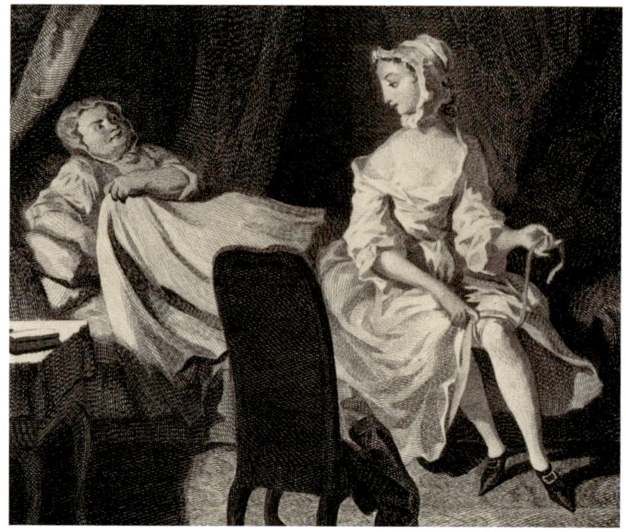

61 'Pamela', Plate 7: *Pamela undressing herself*, detail

offering the promise of an enjoyable, guilt-free sexual encounter. In the seventh scene of 'Pamela' (fig. 61), Highmore presents an equally alluring image of a young female in a state of undress. As seen in Hogarth's image, this lovely girl is accompanied by a grotesque female servant, whose presence increases, still further, the allure of the young woman. It also echoes the pairing of prostitute and 'bawd' or brothel madam. In the novel, Pamela acknowledges the terrible irony of her situation in a declaration at the beginning of her 'imprisonment' by Mrs Jewkes: 'So I find I am got into the Hands of a wicked Procuress'.[33] Later, and prior to the second attempted rape, Mrs Jewkes announces to a horrified Pamela, 'I am a *Jezebel*, and a *London* Prostitute'.[34] Soon after this, Mrs Jewkes directly assumes the role of a Mother Needham figure, overseeing the initiation-rape of Pamela, when she declares to Mr B., 'What you do, Sir, do; don't stand dilly-dallying. She cannot exclaim worse than she has done. And she'll be quieter when she knows the worst.'[35] Richardson's allusions to prostitution give license to Highmore's treatment and visual conceit. Highmore places his Pamela in a posture and gesture of undressing that echoes the prostitute seated in

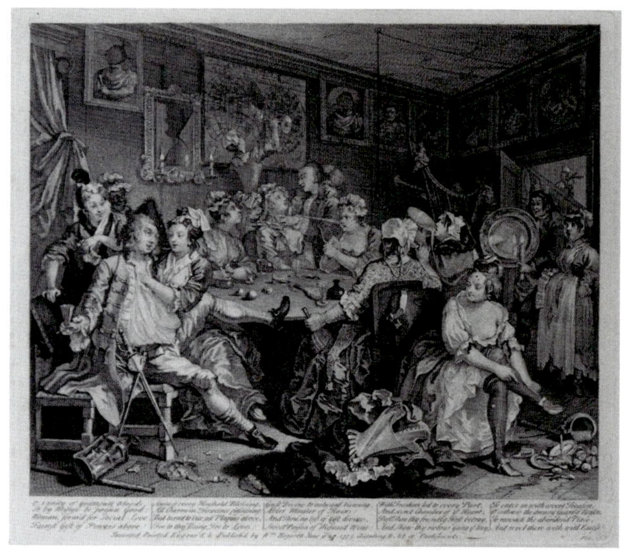

62 William Hogarth, 'A Rake's Progress', Plate 3: *The Rake at the Rose Tavern*, 1735, etching and engraving, 350 x 404 mm, The Garrick Club, London

the right foreground of the third scene of 'A Rake's Progress' (fig. 62), reminding the viewer of a parallel existence for both the male and female protagonists in Richardson's story – should, that is, Mr B.'s perverse designs upon Pamela prove successful. It might also stress that the crucial factors that separate Pamela from Moll – and therefore the course of their histories – is the former's moral strength, religious conviction and education.

Therefore it can be argued that the display and promotion of Hogarth's three series at precisely the same time as Highmore's 'Pamela' would have acted as a timely reinforcement to the visual references to Hogarth's prints within Highmore's scenes, as well as to the broader connections that existed between the respective narratives and main characters. After all, contemporary print collectors in general, and those interested in Hogarth's modern moral subjects primarily, were Highmore's target audience. Further, Highmore acknowledges the perceived ambiguities of Richardson's novel through his inclusion of the sexually charged scenes incorporating allusions to Hogarth's works and, in particular, to his contemporary portrayal of harlots. When placed in the context of the twelve selected images, they more emphatically demonstrate the extent of Pamela's torment and the terrible price of surrender.

'A-LA-MODE'

As discussed, the Hayman-Gravelot illustrations indicated the potential of *Pamela* for a commercial print venture. They also offered a contemporary response to Richardson's novel by a French artist.[36] There is a striking similarity between Mr B.'s clothing in the painted version of the second scene from Highmore's 'Pamela' (fig. 63) and Gravelot's small 'conversation' *Le Lecteur or the Judicious Lover* (fig. 64). If Highmore's image post-dates that of Gravelot, it could be an example of Highmore utilizing the French artist's style and compositions, in this instance to highlight the contrasting behaviour of the male 'lovers'. The idea that Highmore was a follower of Gravelot, rather than simply a contemporary, has long held currency, particularly in regard to his 'Pamela' series: as Ellis Waterhouse argued, the 'importance of Gravelot ... can hardly be overestimated in this connexion'.[37] Later, in a more general assessment of Highmore's output, Waterhouse observes that, before Thomas Gainsborough 'it was Highmore who felt this influence most and corrupted it least'.[38]

But, rather than relying so heavily on the mediation of this London-based Frenchman, Highmore's travel and first-hand experience of the Paris art scene in 1734 would have been the key to his knowledge and skill in the use of recent and contemporary French art.[39] In addition to inspecting the *morceaux de réception* viewable at the Académie Royale, Highmore visited the residences of significant collectors of contemporary art, including Pierre Crozat, a patron of Jean-Antoine Watteau, whom Highmore visited three times. He was also invited to a number of artists' studios, including those of the *fêtes galantes* painters Nicolas Lancret and Charles-Antoine Coypel.[40] Meanwhile, there was a buoyant trade in London for recent and contemporary French paintings, through dealers such as Francesco Geminiani (1687–1762), and engravings were also in plentiful supply. From 1723 to 1735, for example, Jean de Julienne (1686–1766) published hundreds of engravings by, among others, François Boucher (1703–1770) after paintings and drawings by Watteau.[41] Therefore Highmore would have been well aware of the gamut of fashionable French visual culture, which he could adapt and use in his own work.

Returning to the second scene in the summerhouse, Pamela has been interrupted, yet again, in a private moment. A textile is shown tumbling on to the floor, which signals a sudden movement has just occurred. The engraving's text states that the picture shows 'Mr. B expostulating with Pamela in the Summer house after some liberties taken'. That the figures have travelled the distance from the side of the summerhouse (where the abandoned fabric is lying) to its centre hints at an uncomfortable and unexpected struggle. The initial appearance of courtship or an action akin to dancing – innocent enough and a legitimate reason

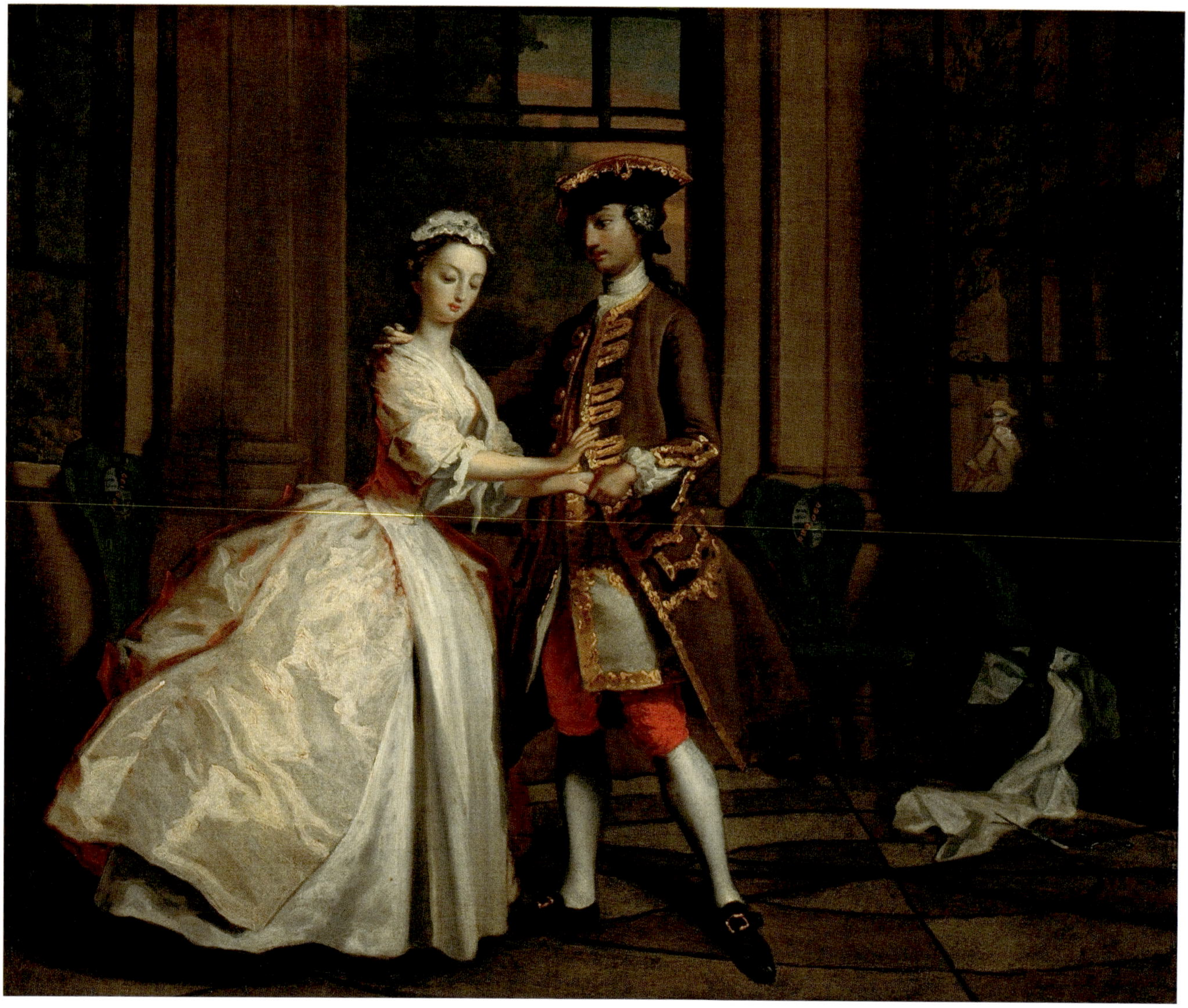

63 Joseph Highmore, *Pamela and Mr. B. in the Summer house,* c.1744, oil on canvas, 62.9 x 75.6 cm, The Fitzwilliam Museum, Cambridge

for unmarried couples to touch – has been infected by gestures that are unpleasant to the recipient and jarring to the contemporary early Georgian viewer. Mr B. holds Pamela's shoulder with one hand, which allows his arm to encircle her back, while tightly grasping, rather than gently holding, her hand with the other. This is balanced by her other hand raised both in surprise and objection to his aggressive and inappropriate behaviour. The lift of her skirts suggests a swinging motion, as if she has been reeled around into her current position, again hinting at the misuse of acceptable social interaction.

As has been thoroughly explored in regard to Watteau's *fête galante* scenes (fig. 65), socially unthreatening behaviour is often juxtaposed within the paintings with incorrect conduct or *faux pas*.[42] The central focus of the image might be a couple dancing in an appropriately respectful and graceful manner while, within the extended company, a man touches a woman in an inappropriate way, causing her to flinch

undressing by French contemporary artists. That Highmore intentionally created a sexually charged image becomes evident from an oil version of this scene (fig. 5.34) which was sold by Christie's in 1954. It is recorded as the same size (25 × 30 in.) and format as the other painted scenes and is therefore certainly Highmore's original idea for the composition.[43] The basic composition is identical with the final version – the partially hidden Mr B. to the left, Pamela seated centrally and turning to Mrs Jewkes in the bed to her right. Yet, in the second version, Pamela is fully clothed, a thick dark shawl partially covering her white chemise or shift and a full-length skirt obscuring her legs. This reduces, significantly, the sense of vulnerability in the central figure, along with the sexual menace so vital to the course and purpose of Pamela's history. Highmore clearly had second thoughts and arrived at a depiction of Pamela that was more audacious and sensationalist,

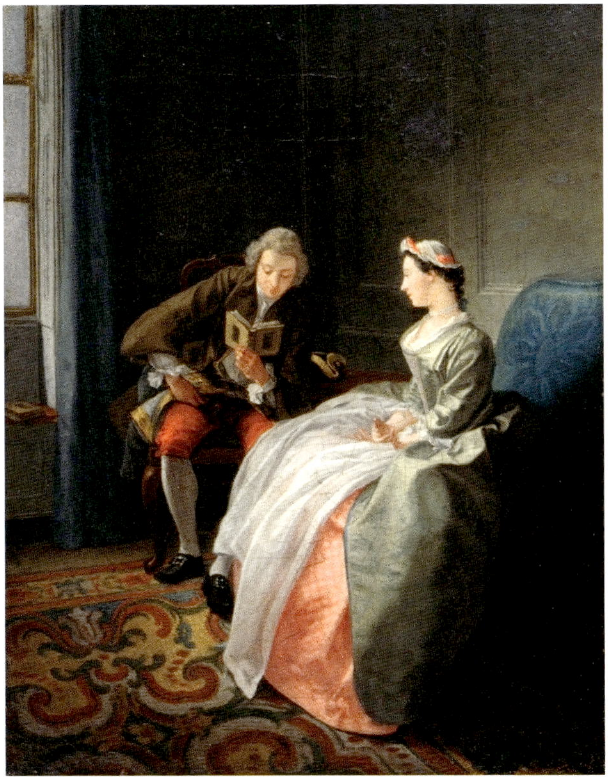

64 Hubert François Gravelot, *Le Lecteur or the Judicious Lover*, c.1745, oil on canvas, 31.1 x 23.4 cm, Marble Hill, English Heritage

and sometimes visibly to remonstrate through an unguarded look and gesture (e.g. the figures to the left of the central female). This event is witnessed, ignored or remains unseen by others close by. In the second scene from *Pamela*, Highmore has conflated these two motifs. The *faux pas* together with the flinch in reaction are grafted on to the 'innocent' dance-like postures apparently displayed by the two main figures. Highmore also introduces a third figure, Mrs Jervis, seen through a window to the left (which the text draws attention to), who, like a character from a Watteau painting, might be close enough to hear or even see the struggle in the summerhouse – and therefore intervene – but, instead, faces away from it.

As observed, in the seventh scene (fig. 66) Highmore's composition cleverly alludes to Hogarth's 'Harlot' and 'Rake'. At the same time he draws direct parallels with erotic scenes of women dressing and

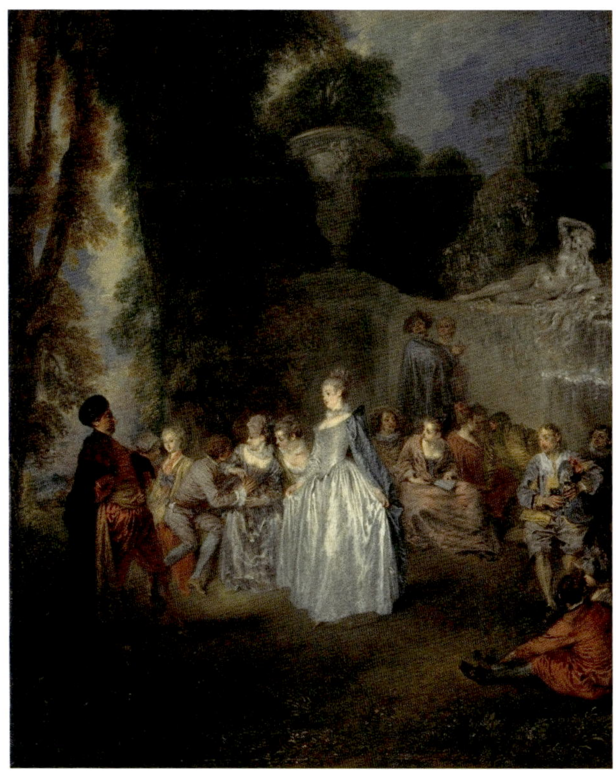

65 Jean-Antoine Watteau, *Fêtes Vénitiennes*, 1718–19, oil on canvas, 68.3 x 57.8 cm (framed), Scottish National Gallery, Edinburgh, Bequest of Lady Murray of Henderland, 1861

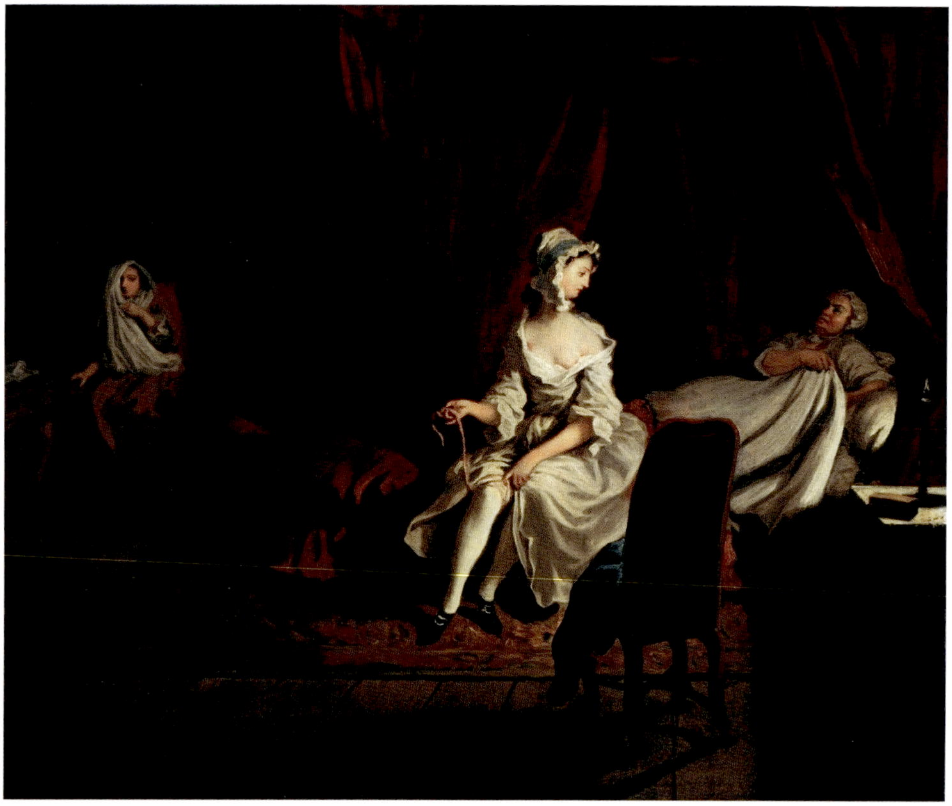

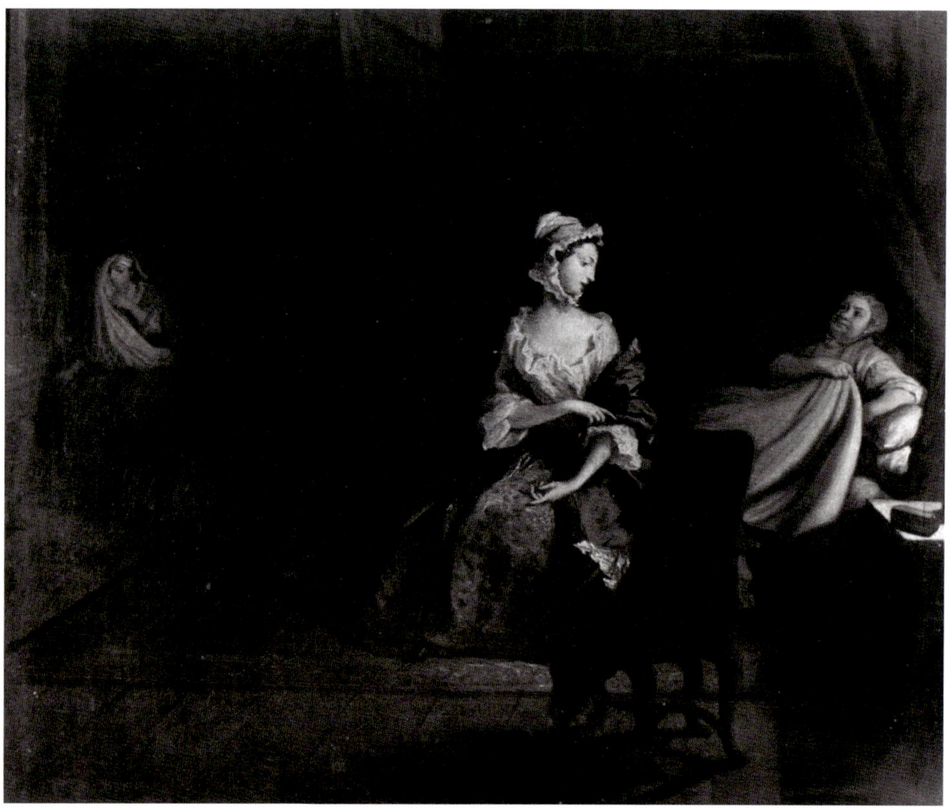

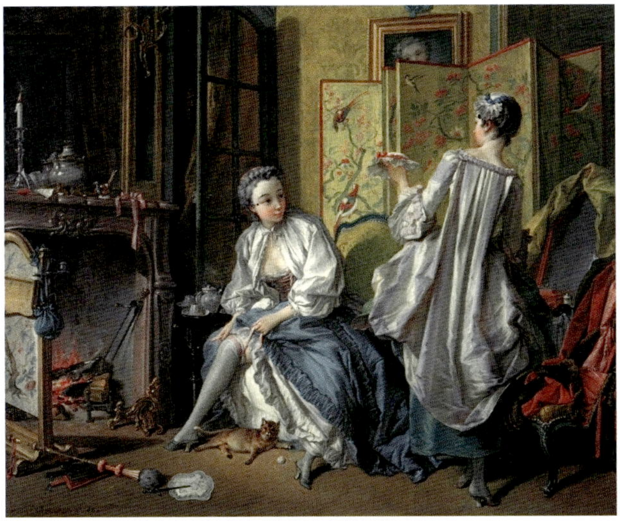

68 François Boucher, *Lady fastening her Garter or La Toilette*, 1742, oil on canvas, 52.5 x 66.5 cm, Museo Thyssen-Bornemisza, Madrid

FACING
66 Joseph Highmore, 'Pamela', VII, *Pamela in the Bedroom with Mrs. Jewkes and Mr. B.*, 1743–34, oil on canvas, 62.7 x 75.7 cm, Tate

67 Joseph Highmore, *A Scene from* Pamela, c.1744, oil on canvas, 61.0 x 73.7 cm, current location unknown

no doubt with the effect on his studio visitors and potential subscribers – as well as his narrative agenda – foremost in his mind.

The pose of Highmore's Pamela echoes the seated female in François Boucher's *Lady fastening her Garter (La Toilette)*, painted in 1742 (fig. 68). The similarities are most evident in Highmore's canvas version (see fig. 67), where both are facing in the same direction with head turned to the right; are shown tying or untying a garter on the same leg that has been placed forward; and are depicted with their arms similarly positioned.[44] Highmore offers even more exposed flesh than can be seen in the Boucher and, in the painted version, the hint of a nipple. The voyeuristic quality is as strong in Highmore's image as in the Boucher: unlike the Harlot, neither woman engages directly with the viewer of the painting and are therefore, at least in Pamela's case, unaware they are being watched. Yet, along with the echoes from Hogarth's 'Harlot' and 'Rake', Highmore is acknowledging the erotic potential in Richardson's story and deliberately encouraging a complex reaction in the painting's viewer. Crucially, Highmore establishes Pamela as a woman that is in every way attractive to men, including sexually. But this fact does not give them license to abuse and defile her. As a result, Mr B.'s sexual attraction for Pamela is understandable and even legitimate. It is his attempt to satisfy his desires by brute force, demonstrably without consent and outside marriage, that is reprehensible and immoral.

Both Waterhouse and later Ronald Paulson offer another French prototype for Highmore's treatment. As Paulson argues, Highmore's images are 'much closer to the contemporary French compositions of Chardin'. He goes on to observe that the 'engravings after Chardin by François Bernard Lépicié, executed between 1739 and 1742, would have demonstrated Richardson's thesis that a maidservant could serve as the principal figure in a work of art'.[45] Engravings after the works of Jean-Siméon Chardin (1699–1779) were readily available in London in the 1730s and 1740s, offering Highmore up-to-date source material for his compositions.[46] At the same time Chardin's paintings were on view in London salerooms.[47] And, prior to this, Highmore would have had the opportunity to acquaint

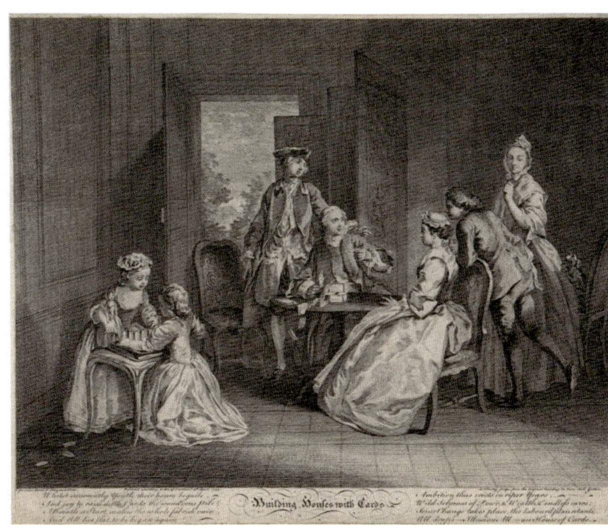

69 Louis Truchy after Francis Hayman, *Building Houses with Cards*, 1743, engraving, 283 x 352 mm, Yale Center for British Art, Paul Mellon Collection

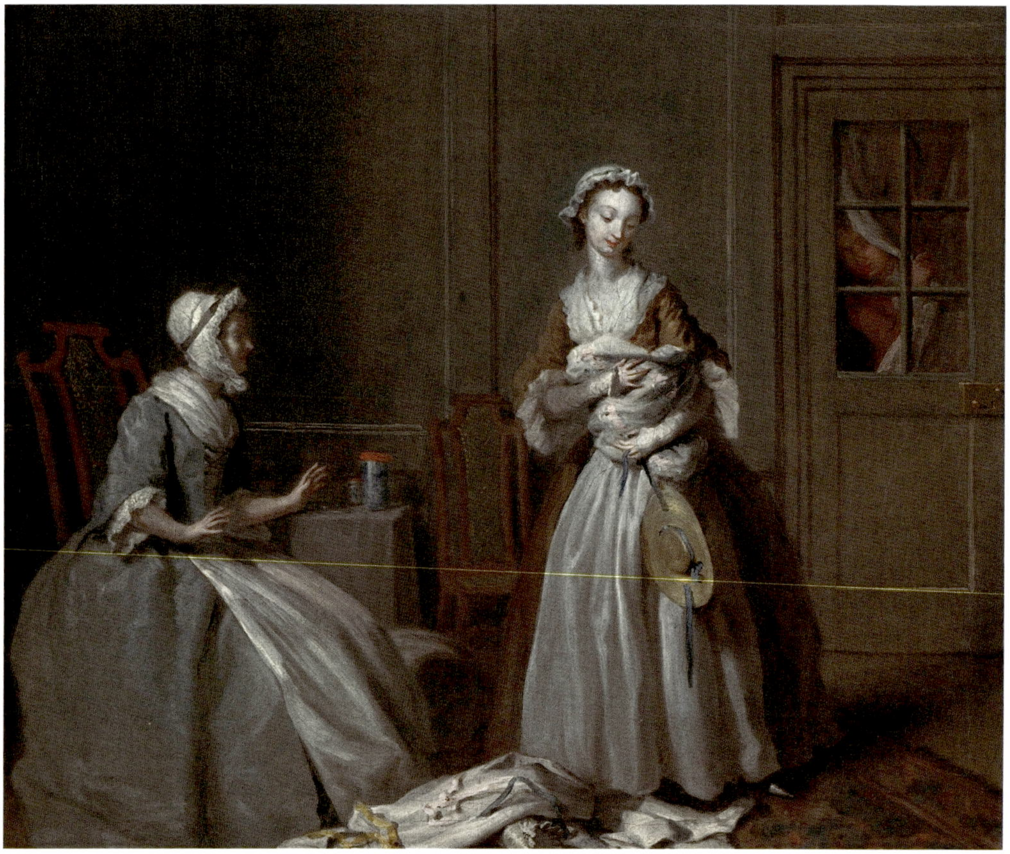

70 Joseph Highmore, 'Pamela', IV: *Pamela preparing to go Home*, 1743–34, oil on canvas, 63.5 x 76.2 cm, National Gallery of Victoria, Melbourne, Felton Bequest, 1921 (1115-3)

himself with Chardin's work while in Paris. In June 1734, Chardin submitted sixteen paintings to the Exposition de la Jeunesse located in the Place Dauphine, a short walk from Highmore's lodgings that summer in the rue Dauphine.[48] Truchy's engraving after Hayman's Vauxhall supper-box painting *Building Houses with Cards* (fig. 69) offers an example of the swift appropriation of a popular Chardin motif by an English artist.[49] It might also explain why Highmore chose Truchy as one of his engravers.

In the fourth scene, Pamela is portrayed in a dignified and restrained manner, despite the emotional turmoil she has experienced in the previous scene. For the first time she is shown, symbolically, unhooped and wearing simple clothing, rather than the elegant aristocratic gifts and 'cast offs' of her deceased mistress.

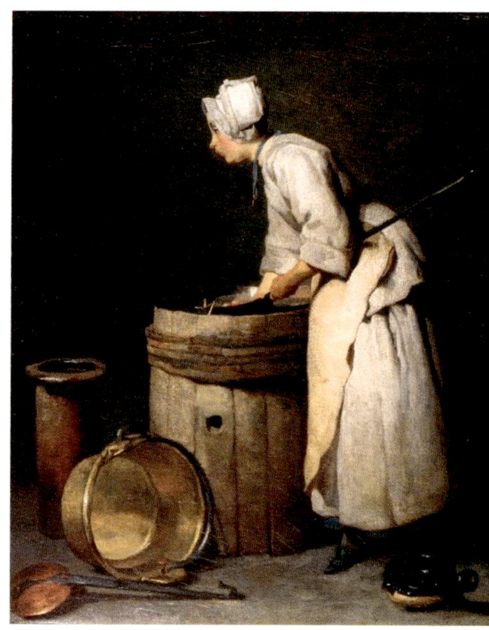

71 Jean-Siméon Chardin, *The Scullery Maid*, 1738, oil on canvas, 45.7 x 36.9 cm, The Hunterian, Glasgow

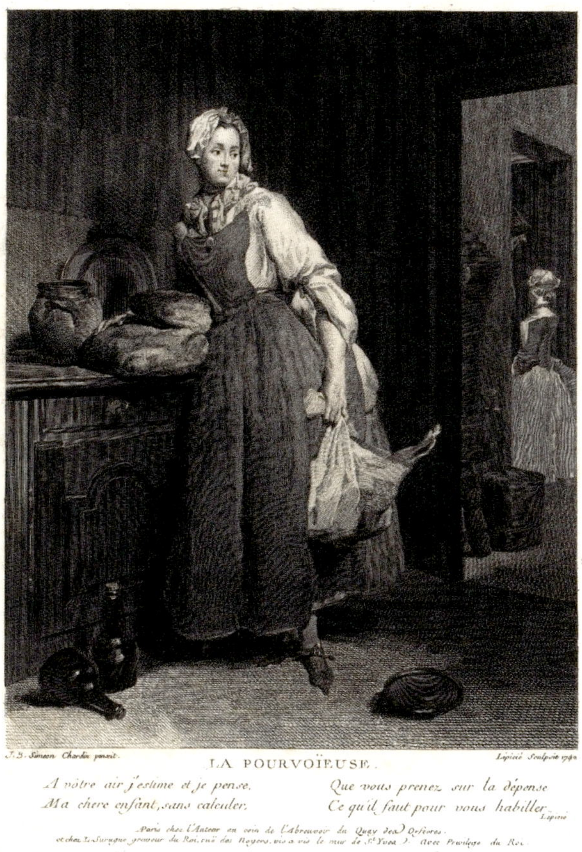

72 François-Bernard Lépicié after Jean-Siméon Chardin, *La Pourvoïeuse* or *La Pourvoyeuse* or *The Provisioner*, 1742, etching and engraving, 375 x 259 mm, The Fitzwilliam Museum, Cambridge

Chardin's images (painted and engraved in turn) of lone or paired servants, as Paulson suggests, would have offered a suitable prototype for this image of Pamela. In the painted version of the fourth scene (fig. 70) the restraint displayed by Pamela corresponds with the reduced tonal palette of white, pale grey, blue and brown – a palette that echoes the subtle modulation of tones in Chardin's canvases (fig. 71). Further, in Chardin's *Return from Market* of 1739, engraved by Lepicié and published in 1742 under the title *La Pourvoyeuse or The Provisioner* (fig. 72), the subject stands in a pantry with a bundle of market goods. She half turns towards the open door, through which is seen a young woman in a boned bodice and full skirt. Her costume contrasts with the more functional clothing worn by Chardin's main figure. Her awareness of this woman appears to have caused her to hesitate and listen. The print by Lepicié includes a text provided by the engraver that is intended either to explain or to project an explanation on to Chardin's image: *A vôtre air j'estime et je pense/ ma chere enfant, sans calculer/ que vous prenez sur la dépense/ ce qu'il faut pour vous habiller* (From your look, my dear young girl, I reckon and believe that, recklessly, you borrow from the housekeeping what you need to clothe yourself).[50] Pierre Rosenberg has dismissed this sentiment as not only spurious but an undervaluation of Chardin's meaning,[51] and in truth such a negative vision of the servant would have had no relevance to Richardson's *Pamela*. Yet, crucially, it offers a contemporary interpretation that establishes servants' clothing, and particularly the moral as well as financial cost, as a visible point of interest: not only is the 'figure' of the servant established as a suitable subject for art, but also their private concerns, behaviour and morality.

This reading supports the use of such images as models for Highmore's 'Pamela' and specifically for his fourth scene, where Pamela's sense of dignity in poverty is represented by her choice of clothing. Despite Highmore's explanatory text describing Pamela as 'haranguing' during this scene, suggesting heightened passion, this is not evident in Pamela's posture or expression. Instead she stands quietly contemplating her 'precious bundle'. As Rosenberg and more recently Juliet Carey have discussed, Chardin was admired as an artist who expressed the interior life through stillness: the gestures and expressions of his figures are restrained and composed, illegible, encouraging interpretation and story-telling, as seen with the text appended to the Lepicié engraving.[52] Pamela's expression is similarly serene. She gazes down at the bundle she holds so gently it could be a swaddled infant. Only Mrs Jervis's reaction hints at the drama of the event. Highmore has apparently reproduced one of Chardin's scenes of everyday life and then strategically activated some of the figures – Mrs Jervis raising her hands and Mr B pulling back the closet curtain – to herald a transformation from a quietly domestic to an overtly dramatic scene.

In all these examples Highmore is not exaggerating and satirizing the *fêtes galantes* and *tableaux de modes* or gratuitously mimicking the scenes of everyday life, but rather employing the recognizable artistic language of these genres with subtle modifications. It is a more sophisticated and respectful, 'bilingual' approach to French contemporary art, which sees Highmore actively engaging with the language of recent French artistic practice for creative, narrative and compositional reasons. In the first instance his likely intention was to appeal to those British collectors and dealers in French art (including graphic art) who celebrated it as a measure of cultural sophistication. More broadly, perhaps, there was the English/British enjoyment of perceived national difference that such art reflected. And yet, considering the international fame of Richardson's novel and therefore the commercial potential for images deriving from it abroad, Highmore's respectful use of such imagery might also have been intended to appeal to Paris-based collectors and artists. As Michel Polge has observed,[53] 'The success of English novels, which, soon after their publication, were translated into French or produced in bilingual versions, made the English painters who had illustrated them known in France. Among these was the painter Joseph Highmore, the illustrator of Richardson's *Pamela* in 1741 [sic].'[54]

Significantly, the 1743 French edition of *Pamela* (published in Amsterdam) included fifteen of the Hayman-Gravelot designs, re-engraved by J. Punt and P. Yver.[55] Highmore may have been aware of this translation, signalling the potential for his enterprise beyond Great Britain, and therefore supplied English and French texts. That Highmore's engravings were known in France, as Polge claims, is established from an entry under 'Truchi' in the *Dictionaire de graveurs anciens et moderns* published in Paris in 1767, which notes that 'Il a grave conjointement avec Benoît, douze m. Sujets en t. pur le Roman de Pamela, d'après *Highmore*'.[56] Highmore's strategy therefore appears to have involved, at least in part, the conscious and meaningful appropriation of French art to appeal to both a British and a French market. His use of French models was not simply prompted by their exotic and erotic attraction for a British audience. His images aimed to appeal to local and Continental audiences, and on their own terms.

'BETWEEN POVERTY AND RICHES'

The physical context created by Highmore in each of the twelve 'Pamela' scenes is predominantly that of the interior – dressing room, summerhouse, bedroom, parlour. In two instances there are external spaces where the figures are still enclosed – the fifth scene, in the forecourt of Mr B.'s country house, with Pamela contained within the carriage and Mr B. likewise contained within a room on the upper floor of his house, and the sixth scene, in the walled garden. Within all these contexts detail is sparingly used and, in every instance, space is reduced or tightened around the figures and their actions. This combines to focus the eye on their postures and gestures. Equally, the economical use of detail stresses the importance of what Highmore has chosen to include. At no point in the composition is the entire architectural space defined: ceilings, for example, are invariably absent. Meanwhile paintings and furniture are cropped or overturned, textiles and clothing are strewn across floors, and humans and animals stand half in, half out of the frame. Some figures are shown in the process of entering or rushing into rooms, or their recent arrival is signalled by an open door. At other times, acceptable behaviour is cast aside by the unseemly grasping of an arm or a shoulder, or the manhandling of a prone female figure. Sanctuary, whether the dressing room, the summerhouse or the bedroom, is ignored and defiled, a circumstance intensified when a male figure is concealed within the space.

The effect is a sequence of recognizable social scenes, usually depicted as still or settled – as seen in a fashionable 'conversation piece' – but here in varying degrees of instability. What we are observing is not the status quo, but a type of controlled experiment, which, from the outset, disrupts and ultimately transforms entrenched presumptions concerning the social hierarchy and, in particular, the condoning and normalizing of unacceptable behaviour by the social elite. The catalyst is Pamela, who appears at the centre of every scene. It is the defence of her virtue and her deep-rooted love for her fellow human beings that challenges and then defeats her aristocratic persecutors. Further, although Pamela is represented as a servant and therefore 'lowborn', her rigid sense of self-worth in tandem with her articulate and impassioned statements against the appalling behaviour and assumptions of her 'betters' hint at a developed understanding of social issues closer to an educated and therefore empowered member of the 'middling sort'. In this sense, if the struggle between 'vice', as represented by Mr B., and 'virtue', as represented by Pamela, is the dominant narrative thread emphasized by the series, it is supported by a parallel societal battle between the dissipated, godless, uncharitable aristocracy – by whose example an inherently good man, as Pamela herself believes, has been turned into a would-be debaucher of innocent, vulnerable girls – and their honourable, hard-working, god-fearing 'inferiors'.

In his essay 'On Poverty and Riches' Highmore observed: 'There is however a proper medium, between poverty and riches, which is preferable to either in many respects; and principally as such a state is best suited to the purposes of virtue and of happiness'.[57] This is the psychological position, as defined by Highmore, located between the aristocrat and the servant, to which both Pamela and Mr B. ultimately gravitate. He goes on to conclude,

> And every man's and every day's experience confirms the observation, that this rank has not only the best chance of virtue and contentment; but also, that though they have not so much to bestow, as those who are more wealthy, yet, as they are generally more disposed, so they actually bestow more: therefore it is preferable to any other; and though the extraordinary characters of a small part of those in the highest life, and most affluent circumstances, may shew that virtue is not utterly incompatible with riches, yet these examples are so rare, and the contrary so general, as to evince the great danger of being professed of them.[58]

Highmore's essay is accompanied by a quotation from Horace, *Satires*, I, 1. 106–07, '*Est modus in rebus, sunt certi denique fines,/ Quos ultra citraque nequit consistere rectum*' (There is a mean in all things; and, moreover, certain limits on either side of which right cannot be found) and the proverb, 'Give me neither poverty nor riches, but feed me with food convenient for me'.[59]

As his published thoughts set out, what Highmore has chosen to emphasize is (in his opinion) the moral fortitude, religious integrity and charitable instincts of his own class, as represented by the servant-girl Pamela, who is literate, moral, articulate, accomplished, slender, tall, beautiful, that is, a very 'middle-class' vision of a servant (in contrast to the Harlot). This is in opposition to what he perceives as the inherently immoral, irreligious and uncharitable instincts of the aristocracy, among whom the rare virtuous exception simply proves the general rule. He systematically portrays the disruption to the status quo that Pamela's resistance and resilience causes, until balance and order are restored – not, it should be stressed, through a return to the 'old' order, but through a reconfiguration or even reconstitution of Mr B.'s extended familial circumstances and attitudes and therefore, by implication, the social order itself. The text for the twelfth engraving states that this scene leaves Pamela 'in full possession of the peaceable fruits of her Virtue', therefore emphasizing as her chief rewards her status as a mother and, by association, wife and mistress of a household – rather than definably as an 'aristocrat'. This is strengthened by Highmore's blurring of 'middling sort' and aristocratic interiors. The dressing room, bedrooms and parlours, despite existing within Mr B.'s residences, could as easily be located within the town houses occupied by Highmore's social peers or indeed Highmore himself. Recognizably aristocratic architecture, such as the exterior of Mr B.'s mansion in Scene 5, is a seam that runs through the narrative, but one that is flanked, contained and ultimately dominated by the modesty and 'appropriateness' of the architecture of the middling sort.

Highmore's 'Pamela' series therefore needs to be appreciated as a radical and surprisingly

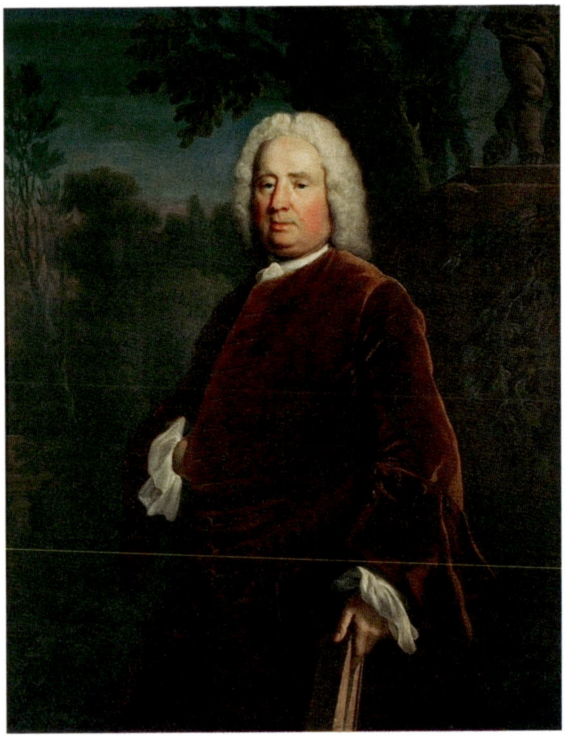

73 Joseph Highmore, *Samuel Richardson*, 1747, oil on canvas, 124.5 x 99.6 cm, Worshipful Company of Stationers and Newspapermakers, UK

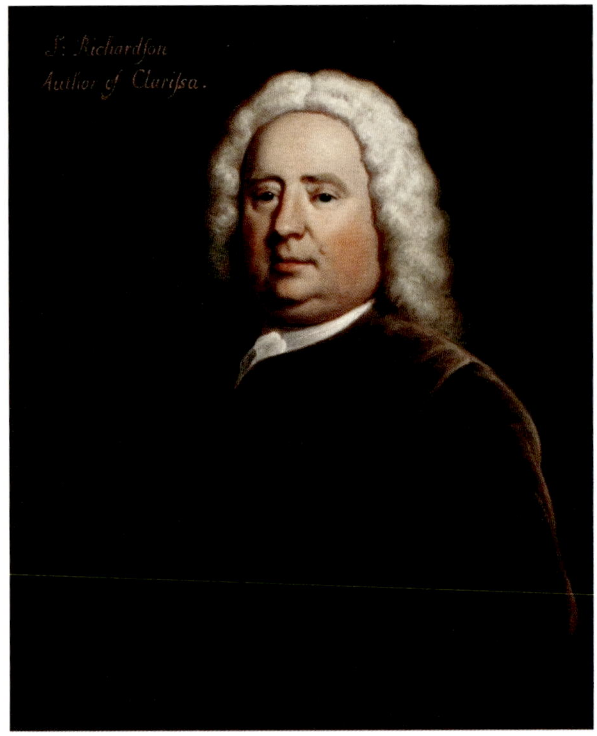

74 Joseph Highmore, *Samuel Richardson*, c.1747, oil on canvas, 76.4 x 63.5 cm, National Portrait Gallery, London

subversive work in its own right – one that seeks to be as penetrating and critical towards the social distinctions, *mores* and behaviours of its time as Hogarth's progresses or 'Marriage A-la-Mode'. Highmore's images are not as obviously loaded with symbols and detail as Hogarth's, nor does he use humour or overt theatricality to assist him in his aims. His method is to assemble and rework the conventions and components of a variety of different pictorial models, which he then fuses into coherent and deceptively simple compositions. It is worth noting that, in responding to Richardson's *Pamela* as, and through, high art, Highmore produced the first such visual response to a contemporary work of English fiction. In the 1740s the novel was still a new art form, and it could be argued that Highmore's sophisticatedly appealing images assisted in defining both *Pamela* and the concept of the novel itself as an intellectual rather than frivolous literary genre.

In addition, Highmore's series can be viewed as part of an ongoing movement by the social 'middle ground' to define itself and its developing power through the appropriation and then modification of the cultural trappings of the traditional ruling elite.[60] Through his particular interpretation of Pamela's adventures, Highmore presents a robust, multi-layered and ultimately heroic visualization of this shifting social landscape and evolving cultural identity.

'A CRIME OF THE BLACKEST DYE'

One immediate result of Highmore's 'Pamela' series was the meeting of artist and author. This led to the production of portraits that were either painted for Richardson (fig. 73) and then engraved by James McArdell at the author's expense or commissioned by his admirers (fig. 74).[61] In light of this, it is safe to assume that Richardson was entirely at ease with

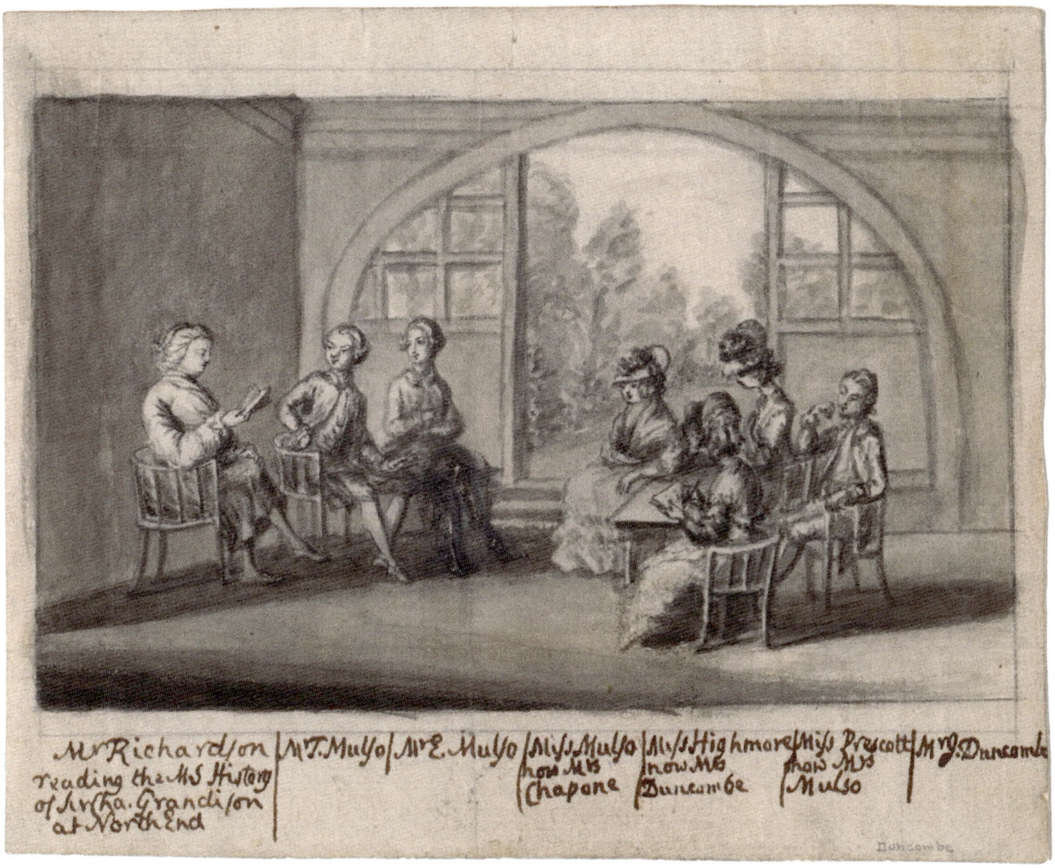

75 Susanna Duncombe née Highmore, *Mr. Richardson reading the MS History of Sir Cha. Grandison at North End*, 1751, pencil with grey wash, 152 x 194 mm, Pierpont Morgan Library, Dept. of Literary and Historical Manuscripts, New York

The scene is set in 'the grotto' at Samuel Richardson's house in North End Road (Selby Lodge) Hammersmith, then a village to the west of London. The author is seen reading aloud the most recent passages from his new novel, *Sir Charles Grandison* (finally published in 1753), for the comment of his young audience (from left to right): Thomas Mulso, Edward Mulso, their sister Hester (the writer and friend of Elizabeth Carter, Mary Delany and Elizabeth Montagu, who later married John Chapone), Susanna Highmore (seen sketching), Mary Prescott (who later married Thomas Mulso) and John Duncombe, Susanna's future husband. The sketch was engraved for the frontispiece of vol. 2 of A.L. Barbauld, *Correspondence of Samuel Richardson*, 6 vols. (London, 1804)

Highmore's interpretation of his work. Indeed, as suggested by Lynn Shepherd, Richardson may have realised that 'the wholesale exclusion of every "warm scene" from his own illustrations had both undermined the reliability of his heroine's account, and caused a radical imbalance within the text.'[62] Therefore Richardson's acquaintance with the artist, which quickly deepened into a sincere and valued friendship between the two men and their families (fig. 75), can be viewed as Richardson's acceptance of Highmore's vision as being one in tandem with his own.[63] Author and artist now united to utilize the promotion of their respective arts to their mutual benefit.

Highmore's 'portrait' of Clarissa Harlowe, the eponymous heroine of the author's second novel, which Richardson described as displaying 'great intelligence, sweetness and dignity'[64] was described within the novel itself – assisting in blurring the lines between reality and fiction. The reference in vol. 3

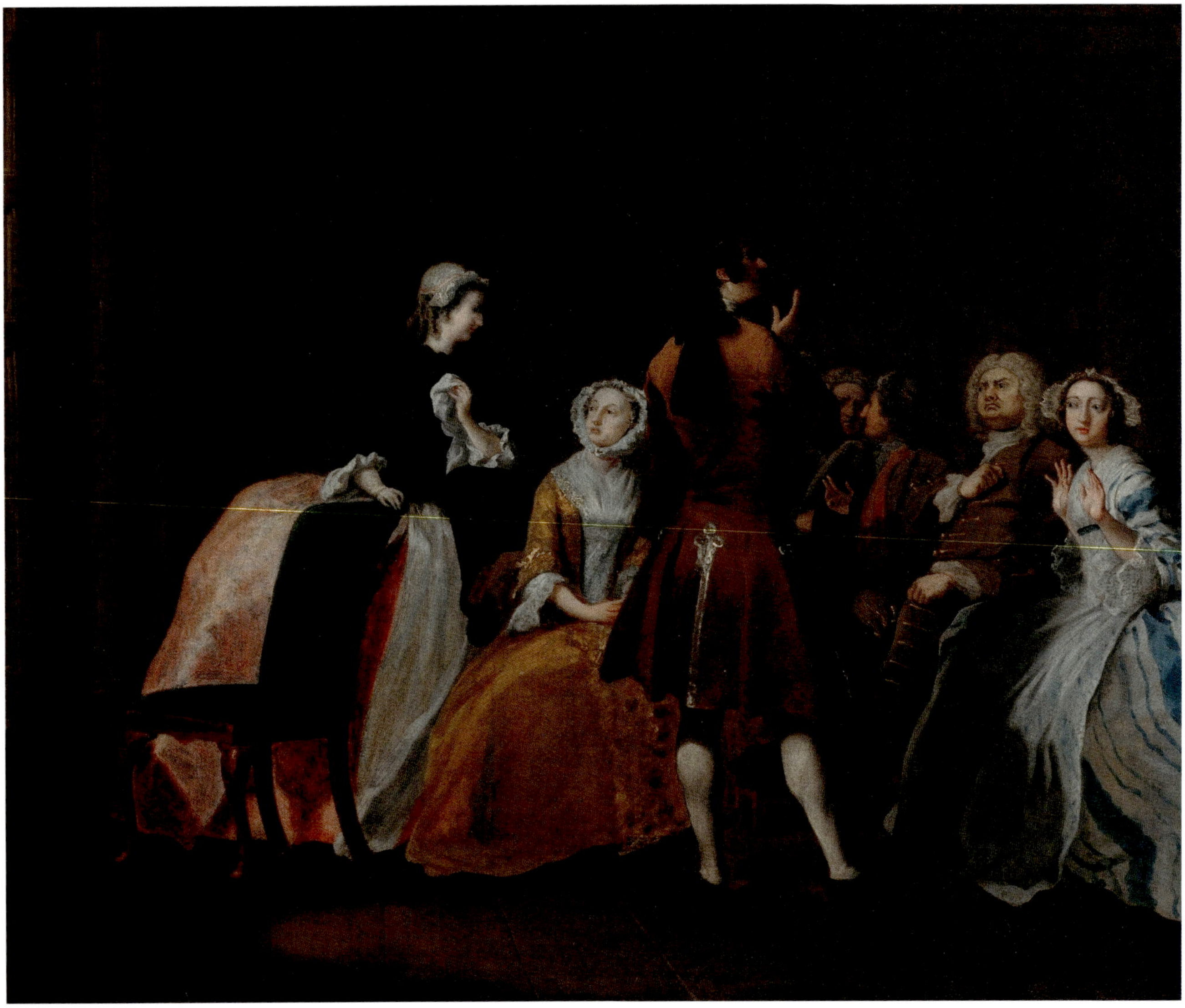

76 Joseph Highmore, *The Harlowe Family, from Samuel Richardson's* Clarissa, between 1745 and 1747, oil on canvas, 64.8 x 78.4 cm, Yale Center for British Art, Paul Mellon Collection

to the 'whole-length picture, in the Van-dyke taste' (of which fig. 77 is an example) that had been 'shewn to every-body ... for your boasted figure' has a footnote that reads: '*This picture is drawn as big as the life by Mr. Highmore, and is in his possession*'.[65] The portrait is later listed among the chattels in Clarissa's will.[66] In addition, Highmore produced a subject painting, known as *The Harlowe Family* (fig. 76), together with a few pencil sketches.[67] The painting is certainly the same mentioned in Highmore's sale catalogue as lot 23, '*Clarissa* return'd Home from Mrs. *Howes*, and accus'd by her Brother of receiving Visits, from *Loveless* [sic]'.[68]

In all but one instance, the focus of the painting and sketches is Clarissa's aggressively bullying brother, whether attempting to force a marriage between the repulsive Mr Roger Solmes and his sister in order to further the family's social-climbing ambitions or reprimanding Clarissa for her association with another

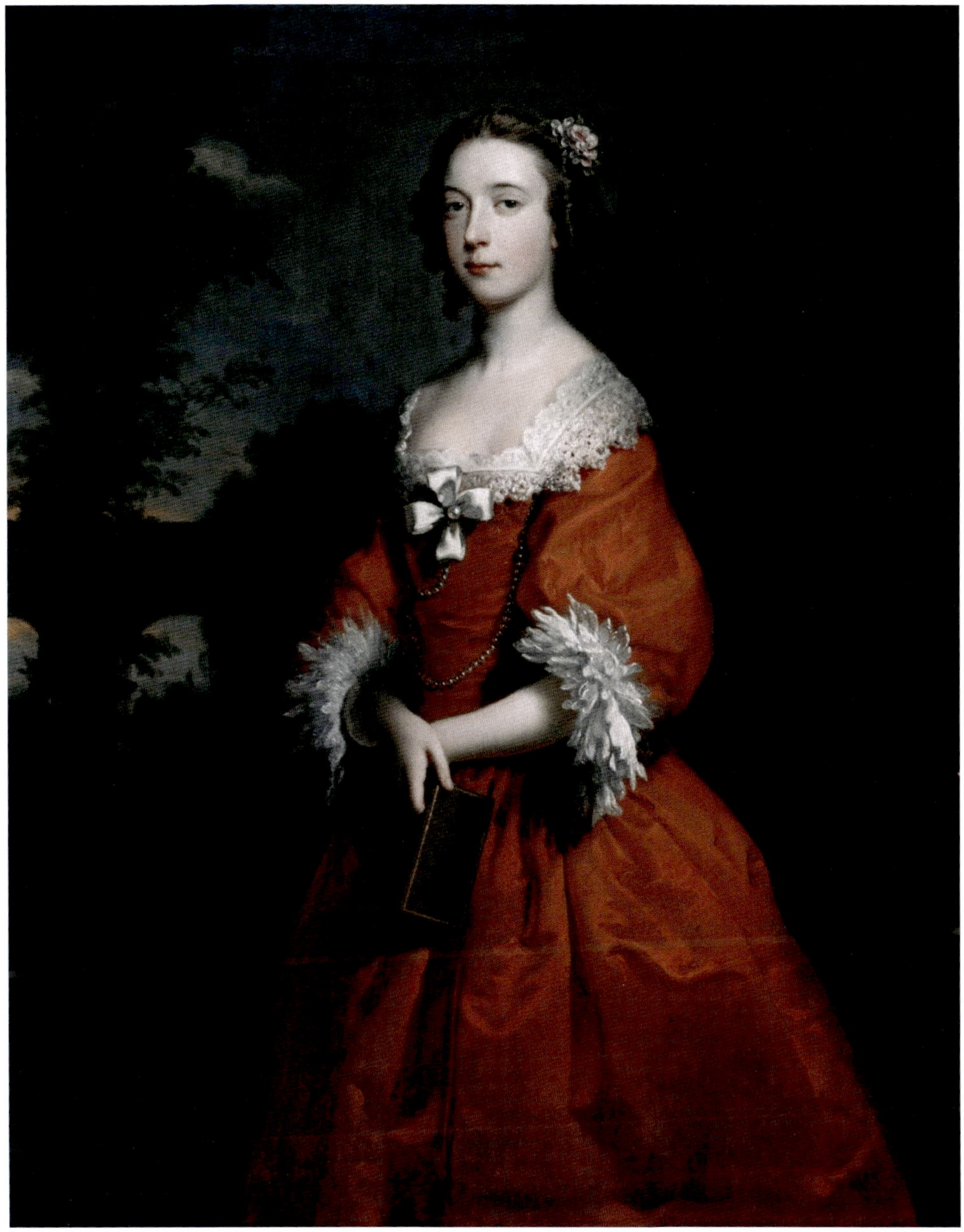

77 Joseph Highmore, *Miss Hamilton*, c.1745, oil on canvas, 127 x 101.6 cm, Detroit Institute of Arts, Gift of Mr. and Mrs. Frederick S. Ford in memory of John B. Ford

Miss Hamilton, dressed in the 'Van Dyck' style, with her light brown hair in ringlets (matching Clarissa as imagined by Highmore in his *The Harlowe Family*) offers a hint as to how Richardson's heroine may have appeared in Highmore's lost portrait of her.

suitor, Robert Lovelace. Clarissa has repeatedly refused to marry Solmes and, in her desperation to escape both this dreaded union and the relentless intimidation of her family, falls prey to the aristocrat Lovelace (pronounced 'loveless'), who turns out to be, in character terms and as his name suggests, Mr B.'s more cynical, dissolute and dangerous cousin. Highmore's canvas portrays the assembled Harlowe family, the central standing figure of James Harlowe acting as the dominant focal point of the group, with Clarissa standing far left.

If we compare this family with *The Vigor Family* (see fig. 33) – another all adult gathering of the same period – the visual signs that brotherly and familial respect and love have all but collapsed become more than evident. Once again Highmore has taken the format and, at first glance, the structure of a conversation piece and strategically activated the figures – whether in gestures of surprise or disappointment, distress or aggression. Clarissa's standing position, which leaves an empty chair within the predominantly seated family group, hints at her imminent and total rejection at their hands. Indeed the description of Clarissa's full-length portrait is from a letter written by her sister, Arabella, in which she describes this painting – Clarissa's avatar – as having been 'taken down' and, along with her sketchbooks, 'thrown into your closet, which will be nailed up, as if it were not a part of the house ; there to perish together: For who can bear to see them ?'[69] Similarly James Harlowe might be mistaken for the elegant figure of William Vigor, excepting, of course, the former's intimidating central presence and snarling expression.

In fully realising one scene only from Richardson's much darker novel – a story where the woman is mentally tortured, abandoned by her family, duped by her admirer, drugged, raped and cursed, eventually succumbing to illness and premature death – it could be assumed that Highmore simply could not find the means to express such levels of degradation and torment in oil on canvas. Equally, Highmore could have concluded, after the effort and expense of his 'Pamela' series, that this single image, coupled with Clarissa's famous 'portrait', was sufficient response to Richardson's latest bestseller, which, in the event, achieved even greater international success than *Pamela*. The significance of the portrait within the narrative, coupled with the footnote, was certainly sufficient to generate the promotion (if he desired it) of himself and his practice. Perhaps friendship with the author had restricted the artist's editorial freedom and therefore, in this instance, his artistic ambitions.

In any event, the success of their mutual promotion can be gleaned from a letter to Richardson, dated to the beginning of 1749, from an anonymous female admirer using the code name 'Belfour': 'May I ask, if there is any such painter as Mr. Highmore, or has he any picture in his possession which we are to suppose was taken for Clarissa? If I live, I propose being in town before I am a year older; and I shall long to see the form he has given her.'[70] The identity of his correspondent was a subject of great fascination and regular discussion between Richardson and Highmore. After an exchange of letters between the author and his admirer, spanning over a year and a half, it was through Highmore's *Harlowe Family* that her identity was finally uncovered. This episode, which can be gradually pieced together through a sequence of increasingly anxious letters between Richardson and the lady, also provides a tantalizing glimpse into an artist's home and studio as a 'public' viewing space.

Richardson had written, in response to the woman's enquiry: 'Mr. Highmore is an eminent painter, in Holborn-Row, Lincolns-inn-fields, the same who published twelve prints of Pamela, of which he has the drawings [sic], and which he had finished before I had the pleasure of knowing him'. In regard to Clarissa's 'portrait', the author states Highmore 'had finished the piece before I saw it, or knew of it, and before Clarissa was printed, having seen only some parts of the work in manuscript. His own imagination was his principal guide.' He confesses that, on viewing Highmore's version of Clarissa, he was ready 'to curse the Lovelace I had drawn'. Finally, he adds, 'Mr. Highmore has also drawn the assembled Harlowes, the accusing Brother, and the accused Sister, on her return from Miss Howe's, as represented in the beginning of vol. I'.[71]

A year later, in February 1750, Highmore was introduced to a visitor in his studio, who made reference to the Harlowe family painting, and, in view of her eagerness and unusually intimate knowledge, the painter suspected that she was Richardson's anonymous correspondent, declaring to his friend, 'I verily believe … that I have seen your Lancashire lady'.[72] In a futile attempt at diversion, the said lady had written: 'What could Mr. Highmore tell you, I wonder? ... So many people call upon him, that I think it would puzzle him to find me out amongst the multitude.'[73] In a later response, Richardson makes the observation,

> Mr. Highmore is a much more lively person, and of consequence more curious than I am; and I believe it is very usual for ingenious painters, when persons whom they know not make a visit to their works, and who are attended by their own equipages, and appear of figure and rank, to be desirous to know to whom they are indebted for the favour done them.

That being true, in conversation with the lady's coachman, Highmore's French servant, John Quiblier, had attempted to tease out the name of the man's master. 'But he being a Frenchman,' Richardson continues, 'so reported the name, and his master so little could depend upon his accent, that he could only be sure that the gentleman was Sir Roger somebody, with a B'.[74]

In ignorance of all this, the lady had arranged another visit, in order for Highmore to prepare the twelve 'Pamela' canvases for viewing – suggesting they were then in store somewhere in the artist's house. Richardson had agreed that, should the lady appear again, Highmore might make a casual comment in her presence to his wife or daughter, enquiring as to when Richardson was next expected at Lincoln's Inn Fields, so that they could judge the woman's reaction. It seems Highmore exceeded his brief by strategically displaying Richardson's life-sized portrait (possibly the half-length now at Stationers' Hall; see fig. 73) in an adjoining room, which achieved the following reaction: '[W]hen I was particularly desired to walk into the next room, I was more than half dead; but revived a little when I found I was only making a curtsey to your picture, for verily I thought I should find you there in person'.[75]

This spectacular reaction, mistaking the image for the man, would have been very satisfying indeed to a portrait painter. In this manner the identity of Lady Dorothy Bradshaigh, whose father-in-law had been in business with Highmore's father, was discovered, much to her initial irritation. However, soon after, Highmore was sufficiently forgiven by Lady Bradshaigh for her to commission the small, exquisite full-length portrait of the author (fig. 78). It can be no coincidence that, in scale and detail, Richardson, for the purposes of the portrait, appears to have stepped into a parlour from Highmore's 'Pamela'. Lady Bradshaigh had written: 'I would chuse to have you drawn in your study, a table or desk by you, with pen, ink, and paper; one letter just sealed, which I shall fancy is to me. Whether sitting or standing, I leave to you and Mr. Highmore.'[76] Highmore has followed this suggestion, but personalized it by adding a portrait within the portrait – the conversation piece of Sir Roger and Lady Bradshaigh in Van Dyck costume by Edward Haytley of 1746 (now in the Museum of Wigan Life).

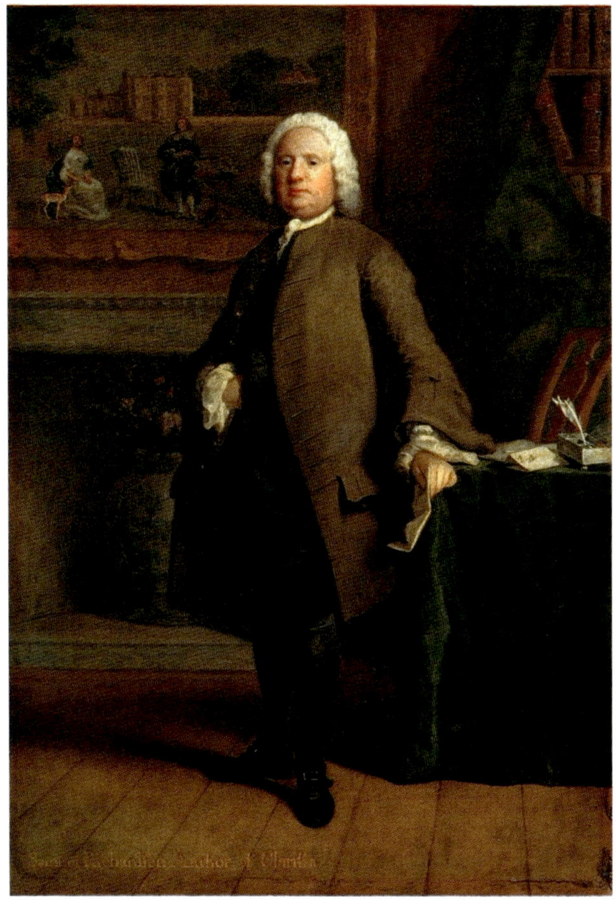

78 Joseph Highmore, *Samuel Richardson*, 1750, oil on canvas, 52.7 x 36.8 cm, National Portrait Gallery, London

Finally, Highmore's close association with Richardson and his heroines may have been the impetus for one unusual action on Highmore's part. Over 1748 and 1749 the former courtesan Teresia Constantia Muilman, née Phillips (1709–1765), published, in short parts, a three-volume memoir under the title *An Apology for the conduct of Mrs T.C. Phillips*. The first advertisement for the memoir appeared in the journal *Old England* on Saturday 16 April 1748, with Part 2 announced on 30 April. Phillips's obituary in *The Gentleman's Magazine*, February 1766, observed that, for a moment, her fate was 'a subject of universal conversation in *England*'.[77] In *An Apology*, Phillips described her rape by the aristocratic 'James Grimes' at the age of thirteen, her abandonment within a few months and subsequent decline into a series of relationships founded on the exchange of money and protection for sex.[78] This publication was not simply a means of generating money for a woman dependent on her wits for survival. Phillips presented to the public a very candid description of the consequences of what she describes as the 'Practice, which is but too common and fashionable, of debauching and ruining innocent young Girls', exposing it as 'a Crime of the blackest Dye' and observing that, as her debaucher has 'now Daughters of his own, let him tremble lest Heaven should punish him; for the Justice of God is generally shown in his Choice of our Chastisements'.[79] It is surely no coincidence that Phillips's publishers, Ralph and Fenton Griffiths, were simultaneously promoting John Cleland's notorious novel *Memoirs of a Woman of Pleasure* or '*Fanny Hill*', the parts becoming available for purchase in November 1748 and February 1749.[80] In a letter dated 15 December 1748, Samuel Richardson himself, writing to the still anonymous Lady Bradshaigh, observes: 'What, think you, has not Mr. Grimes to answer for in the ruin of Constantia Philips, when but eleven [sic] years of age, and abandoning her to the town in two months; if the story she tells be true? What ruins, the consequence of *her* ruin, may not be laid at his door?'[81]

By the time the sixth part of Phillips's memoir was published, concluding the first volume, the revised advertisement dated 16 July 1748 contained the following note: 'N.B. *There is a* Mezzotinto *Print of* Mrs. PHILLIPS *now in Hand, by* Mr. Faber, *from an Original Painting of* Mr. Highmore's, *and will be finished in a few Days*.'[82] The original painting mentioned in each subsequent advertisement was still in Highmore's possession at the time the advertisement was published and it remained in his studio until the sale of 1762.[83] It is currently untraced. Given the mounting furore that accompanied the drip-feeding of Phillips's sensational story, it could be argued that Highmore was not beyond utilizing Phillips's notoriety for personal gain, whether through the advertising of the portrait, its replication via prints – at least two variations are known, both authenticated by Phillips's signature (figs. 79 and 80) – or the encouragement of the inquisitive to view the original in his studio.

However, given the timing of the memoir, Highmore may have had some sympathy for Phillips's personal circumstances. While Richardson was still working on *Clarissa*, Highmore wrote the following in a letter to him concerning the novel's rapist anti-hero, Robert Lovelace: 'Let the Dog be an Atheist or worse, if worse can be; or, at least, say nothing about his religious Sentiments; unless he is represented as an abominable Hypocrite'.[84] Given the tone and content of Highmore's impassioned comments, it could be suggested that Highmore was not simply sympathetic, but self-consciously aligning himself with Phillips's cause: he cannot intercede to prevent either Clarissa's or Phillips's rape, but, in the case of Phillips at least, he can assist her in the exposure of a crime and the redressing of a terrible injustice. Closer to home, Highmore was also the devoted father and protector to a young, unmarried woman – surely an influence on his decision publically to side with Phillips, at some risk to himself. In turn, Phillips no doubt believed her case would be significantly strengthened in the court of public opinion if she had the painter of 'Pamela' and 'Clarissa' as her supporter and image-maker.

Some notoriety by association was no doubt good for a portrait painter's business. When the portrait was finally put up for sale in 1762, it was described as 'the portrait' rather than 'a portrait' of the still living sitter,

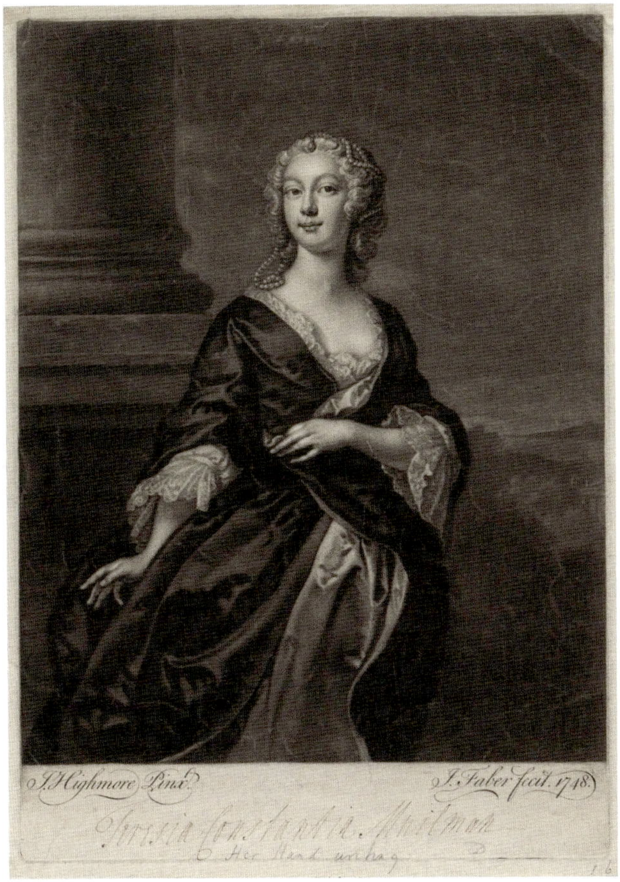

79 John Faber after Joseph Highmore, *Teresia Constantia Muilman née Phillips*, 1748, mezzotint, 366 x 264 mm, National Portrait Gallery, London

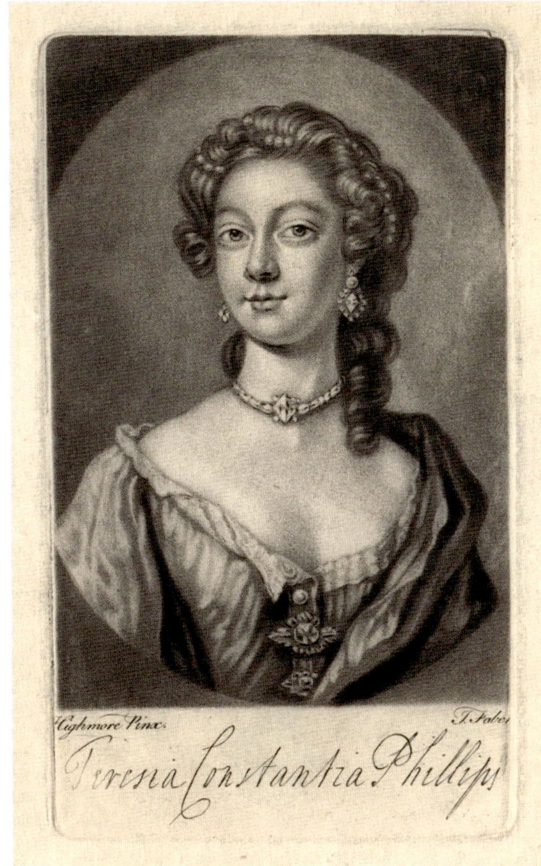

80 John Faber, *Teresia Constantia Muilman née Phillips*, 1748, mezzotint, 164 x 104 mm, National Portrait Gallery, London

in the expectation that her continued infamy would boost the value. Indeed, with the full-length 'portraits' of Richardson's heroines (besides 'Clarissa', Highmore later painted 'Clementina' from *Sir Charles Grandison* of 1753) and the scenes from 'Pamela' and 'Clarissa', this display of popular contemporary literary subjects would undoubtedly have drawn new visitors to the artist's studio, blurring the lines between 'subject' and 'portrait' painting while lending his practice significant topical cachet.[85] Both portraits, along with the twelve 'Pamela' canvases and the Clarissa scene, remained in his studio until the sale of 1762.[86]

Therefore, in 1748, a visitor to Highmore's studio could view the story of the persecuted but ultimately triumphant Pamela, the 'portrait' of the noble Clarissa coupled with a representation of her despicable family, alongside the real-life survivor of an aristocrat's sexual violence, Teresia Constantia Phillips – a thought-provoking, even provocative ensemble. Unsurprisingly, then, Highmore's studio was a notable public attraction, as the satirical poem of 1748, 'The Important triflers' (subtitled 'a journal of pastime a-la-mode, among young-people of fashion') slyly suggests:

> Now and then, for a Frolick, we rove up and down,
> And strole, like wild Creatures, half over the Town:
> Call at *Highmore's*, at *Hudson's*, and step up to *Cock's*;
> See the Lyrichord, Wax-work, Bear, Horse, or an Ox,
> Stop at *Chenevix*, *Deard's*, and, in passing-by, pop
> In the Laceman's, the Mercer's, and the Millener's Shop.[87]

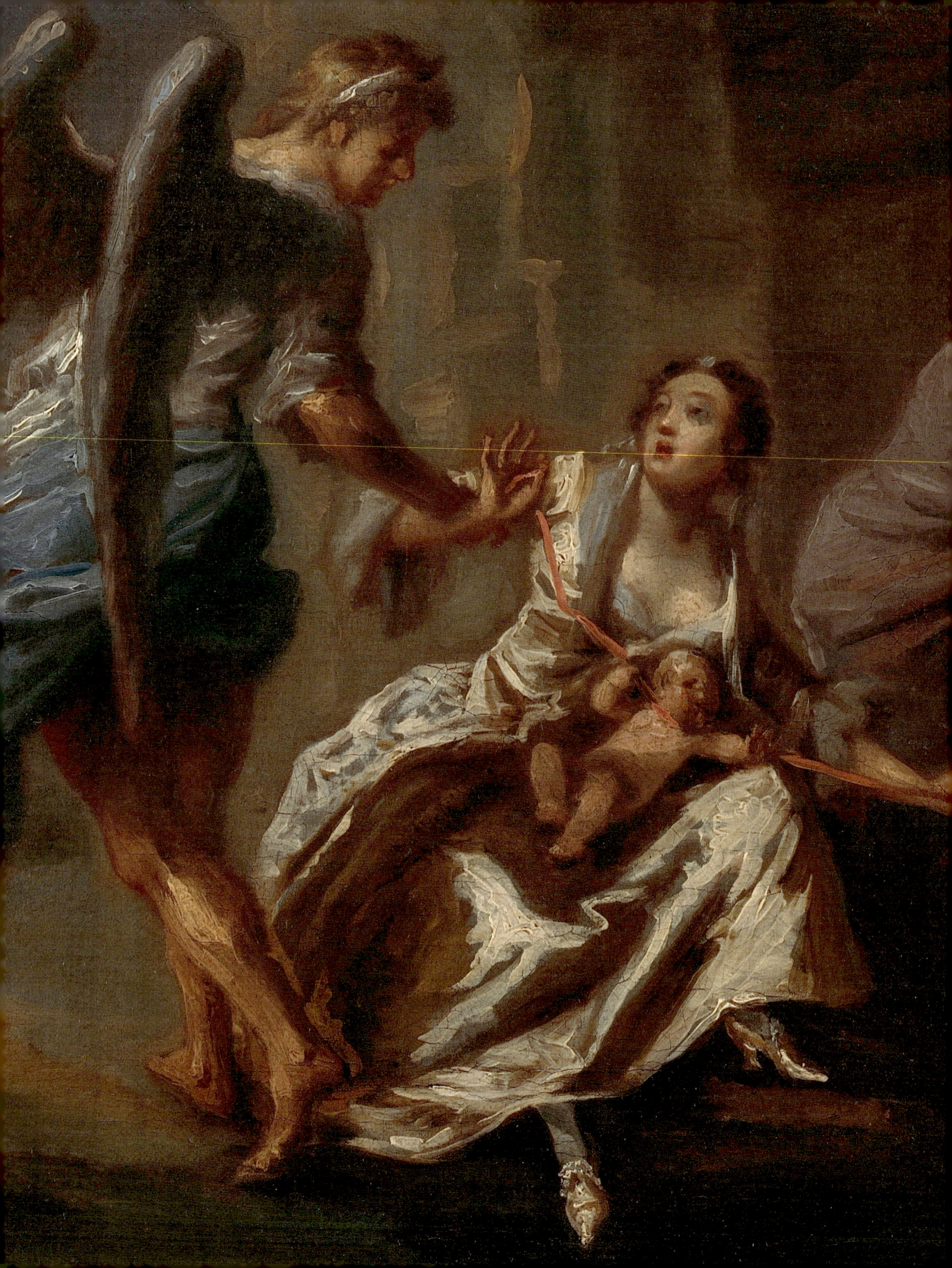

'THE SUFFERINGS OF OTHERS'

The press campaign for 'Pamela' from early 1744 not only advertised this commercial venture, but promoted Highmore's broader ambitions in subject or history painting. Such ambitions were shared by some of his contemporaries, notably William Hogarth and Francis Hayman, but others, like Allan Ramsay, remained content to forge careers exclusively in portraiture. When the opportunity presented itself, Highmore would use his intellect and inventiveness, as well as his sensitivity to character and ability to represent physical form, to push the parameters of portrait painting. *The Lee Family* (see fig. 25) is the prime example. As discussed, this portrait sits at the midpoint between the skill required for 'face painting', the representation of an individual or individuals, and the learning and ingenuity expected of the history painter.

By the late seventeenth century the hierarchy of genres within Western European art practice had been enshrined by the most influential of the state-sponsored art academies, the Académie Royale in Paris, under Charles Le Brun (director 1663–90) with history painting firmly positioned at the apex of artistic endeavour.[1] As the academician André Félibien observed in the preface of his *Seven conferences held in the King of France's cabinet of paintings* (first published in 1705 and here quoted from the first English translation of 1740):

> though it be no small Matter to make the Picture of a Man appear as if it was alive, and to give the Appearance of Motion to that which has none; one who can only draw Portraits, has not as yet attained to this high Perfection of Art, and cannot pretend to the same Honour with abler Painters. He must for that end advance from Painting one single Figure, to draw several together; he must paint History and Fable; he must represent great Actions like an Historian, or agreeable ones as the Poets. And soaring yet higher, he must by allegorical Compositions, know how to hide under the Vail of Fable the Virtues of great Men, and the most sublime Mysteries. He is esteemed a great Painter who acquits himself well in Enterprizes of this Kind. 'Tis in this that the Force, the Sublime and Grandeur of the Art consists.[2]

If portraiture (in its pure form) represented the particular, then history painting dealt with the timeless, the universal – what it was and is to be human. As, on one level, a meditation on matters of life, death and the afterlife, *The Lee Family* consciously entered such philosophical and theological territory.

At the very least, as suggested by Félibien, a reputation in history painting brought greater status to the portrait painter and, by extension, his or her portrait practice. That Highmore strove to achieve this is revealed through four key sources, including Highmore's sale catalogue of 1762, which list fourteen examples of subject pictures, covering biblical, allegorical, mythological, ancient/classical and modern history.[3] Yet only three examples are currently known and all are dateable to the mid 1740s – *The Good Samaritan* of 1744, *Hagar and Ishmael* of 1746 and the oil sketch c.1746 called *The Angel of Mercy*. They are all directly or indirectly connected to one institution, London's Foundling Hospital.

'TENDER IMPRESSIONS'

One of Jesus's most famous parables, 'The Good Samaritan' is recorded in the Gospel of St Luke and tells of a Jewish man who is attacked on the road, stripped of all his belongings and left for dead. Ignored by two fellow Jews (a Priest and Levite) he is eventually assisted by a Samaritan, traditionally an enemy of the Jewish people, who 'had compassion on him ... and took care of him'.[4] At the heart of the parable is the definition of a 'neighbour', and the question of who is a rightful beneficiary of charity and benevolence. Jesus, the narrator, sets up a scenario for the judgment of the listener. He challenges their preconceptions by allowing kindness to be displayed by the victim's 'enemy' rather than his compatriots and asks, 'Which one of these three, thinkest thou, was neighbour unto him that fell among the thieves?'[5] As the Church of England Reverend Thomas Stackhouse (1677–1752) observed in his popular commentary, *The History of the Bible*, first published in 1737, the Priest and Levite 'might therefore be presum'd, even in Virtue of their Office and Education, to have more extensive Notions, and Hearts more capable of tender Impressions ... [yet] he introduces a Samaritan, as acting a different Part, and taking all imaginable Care of this wounded Jew'.[6] Stackhouse concludes, 'the Samaritan was the Neighbour to the Person in Distress, and, consequently, that the Notion of a Neighbour comprehended Men of all Nations, and all Religions whatever'.[7]

Stackhouse's use of such phrases as 'tender Impressions' and 'all imaginable Care' expands on the original text, encouraging his reader not only to admire what the Samaritan does but to consider and then empathize with how and why he does it. It is the unreserved compassion and love toward a fellow human being that directs this charitable act. This is echoed by Highmore's friend Dr Isaac Watts in his *A Preservative from the Sins and Follies of Childhood and Youth*, in which he says: 'Our Saviour in the Parable ... shews that the Jews and Samaritans, how much soever they differed in other Things, should look upon one another as Neighbours, to do all Offices of Kindness to each other'.[8]

Given the source of Highmore's subject, his interpretation would have been shaped, at least in part, by his Christian faith. After his retirement, Highmore published essays on theology and related subjects, including *Observations on a pamphlet, entitled, "Christianity not founded on argument"* (1765), written under the provocative sobriquet 'a Christian freethinker'.[9] Here he argues that Christianity can be defended as reasonable only if those defending it 'content themselves with asserting, and maintaining pure, original Christianity, in its primitive simplicity, without any human additions'.[10] The 'human additions' he specifies as, effectively, the mechanisms of organized religion, particularly but not exclusively the Anglican and Roman Catholic Churches – 'weak and inconsistent systems, creeds, articles and catechisms which cannot be authorised, or supported by Scripture'.[11] He continues, 'If it be asked, on what then does the evidence of Christianity depend? the answer will be, on the Scriptures of the Old and New Testament, but especially the New'.[12] This focus on the primary sources of early, 'primitive' Christianity, specifically the Old and New Testaments, would have had important implications for Highmore's approach to the representation of biblical narratives, and potentially subject painting as a whole. It is clear, as already seen with his approach to Samuel Richardson's *Pamela*, that close personal study and analysis of the key 'original' texts were the foundation of Highmore's creative process. This would be developed and refined, through personal inclination as well as professional training, by the scrutiny of relevant artistic precedents and – perhaps more importantly – by the intended physical setting of the image in question. Through such a method, again as seen with 'Pamela', a fresh and complex approach to the story might emerge.

In 1744 Highmore completed his painting on the subject of the Good Samaritan, a commission for John Sheppard (1675–1747) of High House, Campsey or Campsea Ashe in Suffolk.[13] At exactly the same time, Highmore introduced the Good Samaritan theme into the first engraving and canvas of his 'Pamela' series (see figs. 34 and 54). This was the artist's own invention, perhaps inspired by the Sheppard commission. Although the precise details are unknown, the 1883 sale, as Elizabeth Einberg discovered, of the contents of the essentially Victorian High House – Sheppard's seventeenth-century home had been severely damaged by fire in 1865 – contained an unattributed lot 834, '*The Good Samaritan*' followed by lot 835, '*Pair – Hope and Charity*'.[14] The three pictures, which collectively represented two of the theological virtues ('Faith' being the third) were listed as hanging in the vestibule. As Einberg suggests, Sheppard's house may have had a private chapel and these three paintings, *The Good Samaritan* flanked by the panels of *Hope* and *Charity*, might therefore have formed the triptych altarpiece.[15] As a private commission, Highmore's painting was certainly intended to be an intimate, personal object. If it once formed part of an altarpiece, then the canvas would have been commissioned and therefore conceived as a spiritual image, intended to encourage its audience to follow the virtue represented.

At some time, possibly as part of his research, Highmore visited William Hogarth's recently completed large-scale painting on the Good Samaritan theme at St Bartholomew's Hospital (fig. 81). A sketch by Highmore from the Highmore Family Gift (fig. 82) follows the Hogarth composition closely, including the idiosyncratic detail of the dog licking his own hind leg. In both Hogarth's canvas and Highmore's sketch the first half of the parable has been compressed to include the Samaritan tending the victim and the figures of the retreating Levite and Priest in the background. However, closer inspection of Highmore's sketch reveals that he has already begun to modify Hogarth's composition, creating a more dynamic pose for the Samaritan and adjusting the location or posture of the other figures, including the dog and horse. By the time Highmore composed his own canvas, he had abandoned Hogarth's composition altogether, along with the specific moment from the parable that Hogarth had chosen. This suggests that the intention and therefore effect of Highmore's painting is crucially different to other versions of the parable, including that by Hogarth.

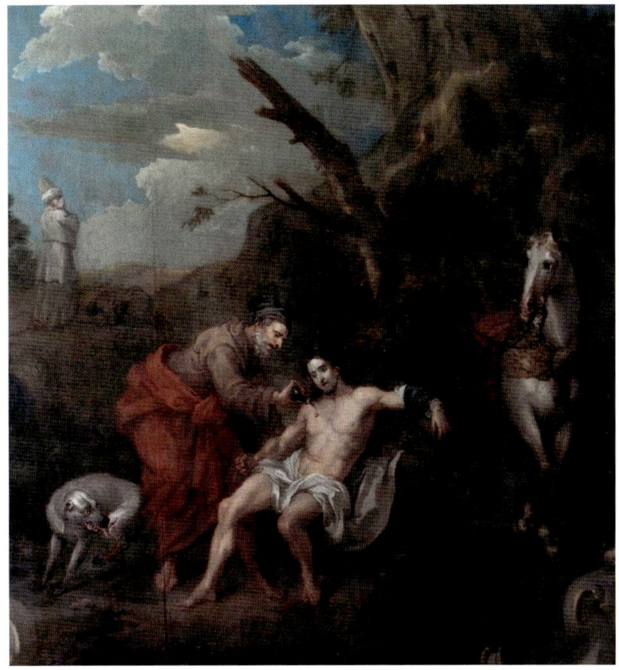

81 William Hogarth, *The Good Samaritan*, 1737, oil on canvas, 508 x 418 cm, St Bartholomew's Hospital, London

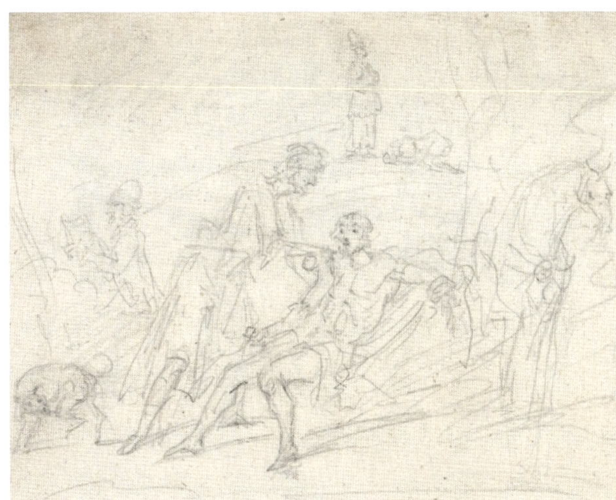

82 Joseph Highmore after William Hogarth, *The Good Samaritan*, date not known, graphite on paper, 83 x 133 mm, Tate

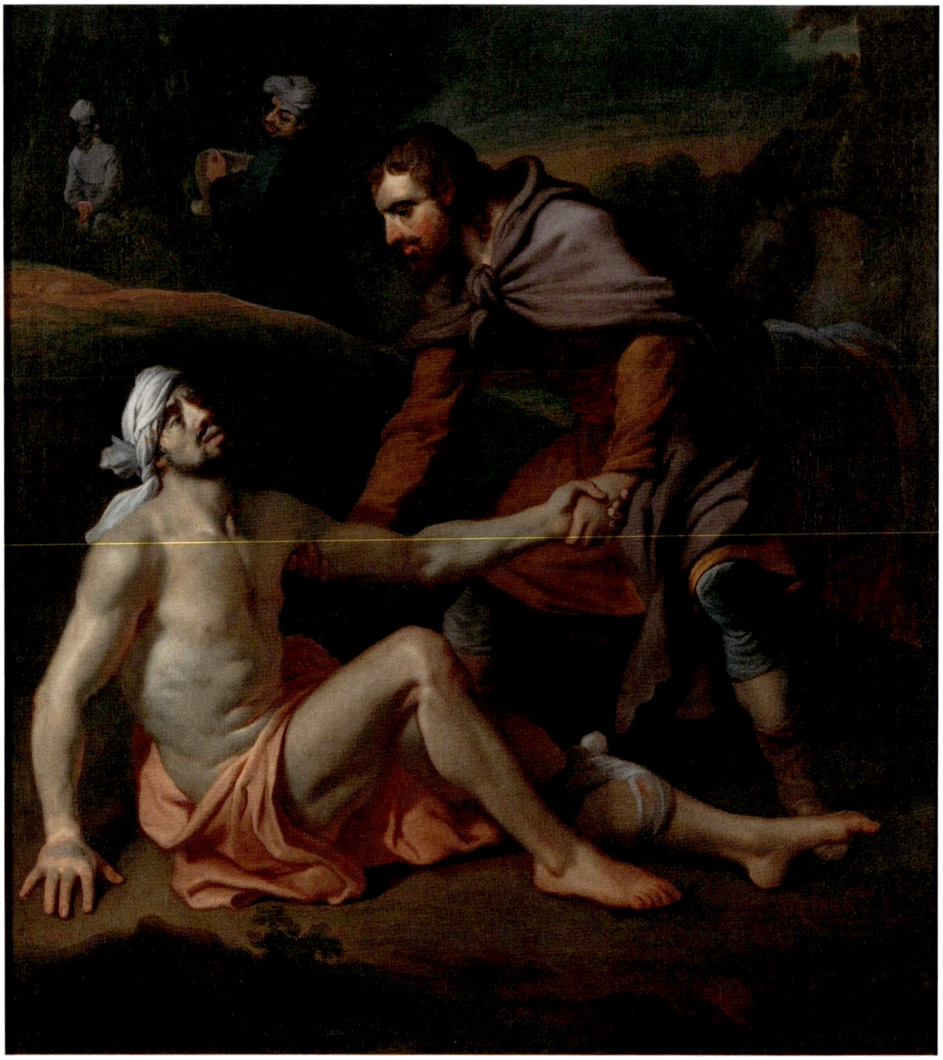

83 Joseph Highmore, *The Good Samaritan*, 1744, oil on canvas, 159.5 x 144.8 cm, Tate

Highmore's composition (fig. 83) is very simple, with few distractions from the central narrative and the two key figures. He has included the Samaritan's horse, the Priest and the Levite but only as supporting details. Highmore's Samaritan has physical features that separate him from the other figures, specifically the reddish colouring of his hair, in line with a key element of the parable.[16] Highmore chooses the moment after the Samaritan has bound the wounds of the victim and is assisting him to rise to his feet. The Samaritan leans forward holding the man's left hand while supporting him under his upper arm. With his legs braced and eyes fixed on his companion, he pauses. The wounded man has placed his right hand on the ground, fingers spread, and is beginning to push up: his anxiety and pain is signalled by his knitted brows and open mouth. In contrast, the Samaritan is reassuringly calm, staring upon his companion's face with purpose and concentration.

Everything is intimated through expression, gesture and touch. There are three key gestures within the composition, the downward tilt of the Samaritan's head; his right hand, gently but firmly supporting the victim's upper arm; and their clasped hands to the centre right. This forms a concentration of interlinked hands and arms at the centre of the canvas, reflecting the practical help the Samaritan has chosen to give, as well as the tenderness that is evident in the biblical text but given greater emphasis in contemporary theological writings.[17] The Samaritan's earnest gaze, which is not returned by the victim, suggests the selflessness of the truly benevolent act. His concentration is on the recipient rather than himself and no direct response is required or expected. Yet, within the suspended action represented by Highmore, there is a feeling that the Samaritan figure, the giver of charity, requires some effort on the part of his companion: concern, assistance and even love are willingly offered, but the recipient must also help himself.

In concentrating on the tending of wounds, Hogarth had placed the story firmly in the arena of practical charity, as befitted its location within a hospital. The detail of the bloodied bandages that bind the head and leg of Highmore's victim acknowledge the presence and importance of such charity. But in setting the action a stage later – that is, after the wounds have been bound – Highmore shifts the focus towards a form of fellow feeling, 'love of mankind', that transcends social, religious and even racial differences, which chimes with the theological writings analysed earlier. He is therefore responding to the spirit and the letter of the parable.

'THE TENDERNESS FOR CHILDREN'

In 1739, after decades of debate, London's 'Hospital for the Maintenance and Education of Exposed and Deserted Young Children' or Foundling Hospital finally received its Royal Charter, and, in tandem with the design of the new building, its potential as a showcase for contemporary British art was conceived. The foundation stone for its permanent home in Lamb's Conduit Fields, just north of the city, was laid in September 1742, with the west wing containing the suite of formal administration rooms, including the Governors' Court Room, completed three years later. Both the 'Pamela' series and *The Good Samaritan* would have been in Highmore's studio at precisely the time when the plan for a series of history paintings was being discussed for the Governors' Court Room, the most ornate and prestigious interior, conveniently offering a visiting Hospital governor or architect evidence of Highmore's ambitions and ability in history and subject painting. However, Highmore's inclusion, along with William Hogarth, James Wills (fl. 1740–47) and Francis Hayman, among the four artists recruited to produce these history paintings, was clearly at odds with the focus of his career to date, portraiture (fig. 84). As George Vertue noted on seeing Highmore's contribution for the Court Room scheme, *Hagar and Ishmael*, in the artist's studio, 'it promises much and shews that his Genius is not so confind, but it may extend it self in that branch of painting with due commendation – as painter of History if he coud meet with suteable incouragement'.[18] It appears that among the broader art community the notion of Highmore as a history painter was a recent and novel development. Yet Vertue also offers an encouraging contemporary opinion regarding Highmore's future career in the genre.

As a founding governor, William Hogarth had established a close association with the Hospital from its inception. He designed the institution's 'arms', the headpiece for the fundraising power of attorney or 'subscription roll', and even, it is thought, the children's red and brown uniforms. Traditionally it has been assumed that Hogarth also not only devised and coordinated the ongoing acquisition, display and promotion of British contemporary art within the Hospital's 'public' spaces but defined the most prestigious painting scheme, located within the Court Room, and the artists invited to participate.[19] This scheme consisted of 'portrait' roundels of London hospitals, including the Foundling Hospital itself, as well as the four large history paintings by Hogarth, Highmore, Wills and Hayman.[20]

The traditional view of Hogarth as the lone presiding genius is certainly an exaggeration. The Hospital's architect Theodore Jacobsen (d. 1772) clearly designed important areas, and particularly the Court Room,

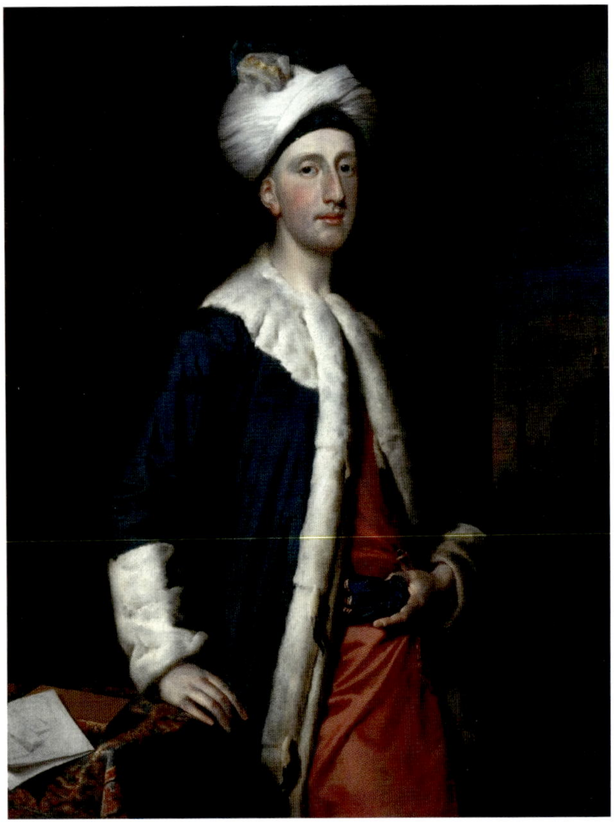

84 Joseph Highmore, *John Montagu, 4th Earl of Sandwich*, 1740, oil on canvas, 121.9 x 91.4 cm, National Portrait Gallery, London

The portrait celebrates the young Earl's recent Grand Tour, which included, unusually at this date, Egypt and the Near East. As a result, Sandwich founded the Divan Club for likeminded gentleman travellers (the official toast, 'The Harem', made in honour of Lady Mary Wortley Montagu). Sandwich is dressed as an Ottoman gentleman, with the famous mosque of Constantinople (now Istanbul), Hagia Sophia, (Holy Wisdom) in the background. His costume is identical to that seen in Andrea Soldi's portrait of the British Levant merchant Henry Lannoy Hunt of c.1733–36 (Tate, T11977)

with some form of painted scheme in mind, as was the case with his earlier work at East India House in Leadenhall Street.[21] Further, the use of hospitals for the encouragement of native artists was not a new concept. In 1731 Daniel Defoe had recommended that selected boys from Christ's Hospital be trained in music, to combat the influx of imported foreign talent, and then noted:

> After-thought. The Scheme, page 16, 17, &c. may be so improv'd to extend to Painting, Sculpture, and other curious arts: Under good Masters the Youths may so improve to make England emulate Greece and Rome, not to mention the Profits that will accrue from their Labours.[22]

Defoe's suggestion that there would be 'profits' (we can assume, from the sale of the art produced within the proposed academy) implies the promotion of public viewing and the encouragement of patronage. No doubt these patrons, the governors and visitors to Christ's Hospital were expected to be one and the same. Here, then, is the commercial germ of the Foundling Hospital's contemporary art collection.

However, regarding history painting, it is certainly the case that since the death of Sir James Thornhill in 1734 – painter of the magnificent Painted Hall at Greenwich and the cupola of St Paul's Cathedral – Hogarth was the only British artist to have had the experience of a prestigious commission within a public or semi-public building. The resulting monumental canvases at St Bartholomew's Hospital (*The Pool of Bethesda* and its companion *The Good Samaritan*, painted 1736 and 1737 respectively) demonstrated that contemporary British painters had the potential and ambition successfully to attempt large-scale works in the historical genre. Yet, as Hogarth's friend Jean-André Rouquet famously declared almost two decades later, 'History Painters have so seldom an opportunity of displaying their abilities in England, that it is surprising there are any at all who apply themselves to this branch'.[23] Because of their limited circumstances for patronage, British artists acquired the habit of making the most of the few opportunities presented to them. The new Foundling Hospital, with its yard upon yard of empty walls and signature spaces, was one such opportunity writ large.

Nevertheless, the Hospital governors had no intention of using financial donations to purchase fine art: the children, rightly, must be the primary focus. As a result, according to Rouquet, the artists collectively decided to donate paintings to the Hospital.[24] Rouquet

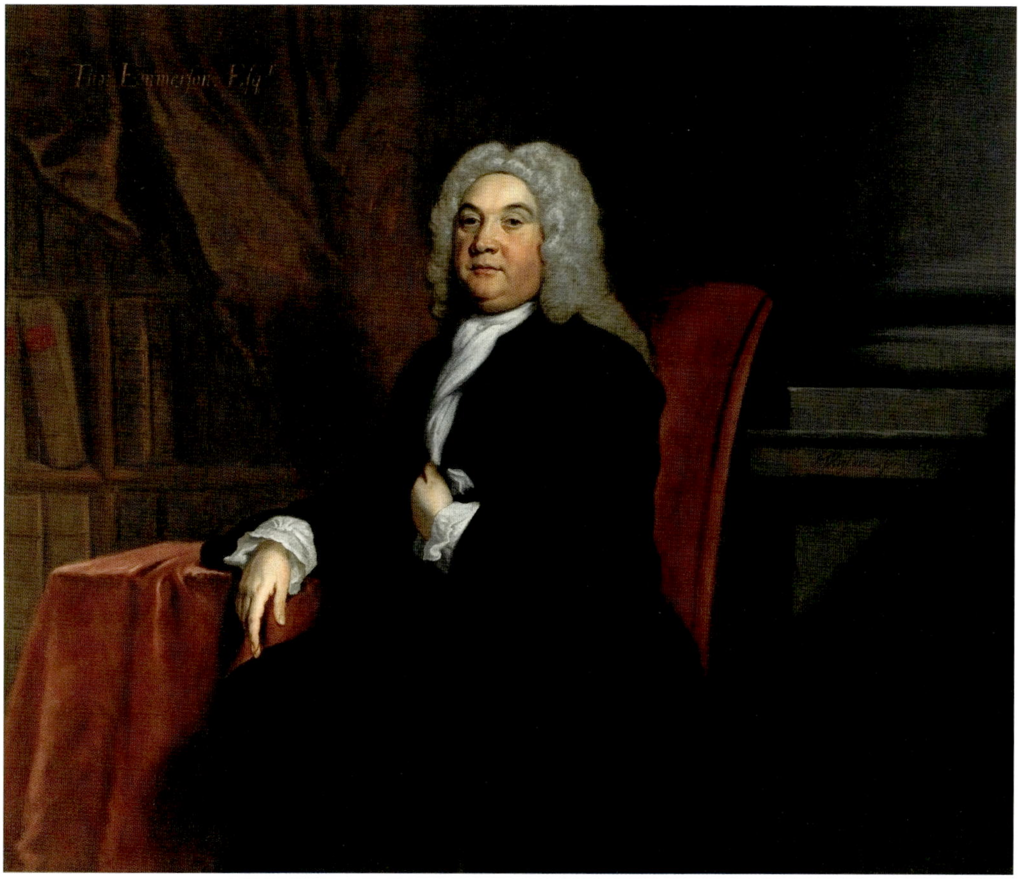

85 Joseph Highmore, *Thomas Emerson*, 1731, oil on canvas, 101.6 x 127.6 cm, The Foundling Museum, London

makes no reference to Hogarth's dominant role in this process, and the first official description of the Foundling Hospital, dated 1749, states simply that such donations stood 'as Monuments of their Charity, and Abilities in their several Arts'.[25] It is worth observing that the charitable gift and the implied personal benefit to the artist donor have been given equal weight within this statement. As commercial artists in a highly competitive contemporary art market, such 'enlightened self-interest' was understandable, even necessary. What is certain is that the opportunity presented by the Foundling Hospital galvanized the artist community into a concerted and unified effort to promote themselves, their national school and the ability of that school in all genres, including history painting, although it should also be noted that, within the variety of genres represented, a significant number of the donated paintings were and continued to be portraits.

The first, in 1740, was Hogarth's full-length of the Hospital's founder, Captain Thomas Coram (c.1668–1751), a portrait where Coram's kindness, as well as his earthiness, grit and resolve – vital traits in his twenty-year battle against inertia and prejudice to establish the Hospital – are all beautifully expressed in the sitter's gentle, alert and weather-beaten face. Highmore's earlier portrait of the sugar baker (a refiner of raw sugar from the plantations of Barbados) and Hospital governor-benefactor Thomas Emerson (of 1731) was also among the donated paintings (fig. 85). Emerson, formerly based in Thames Street (where Highmore had been born) but at his death living in the village of Battersea, left the portrait to the Hospital in a codicil

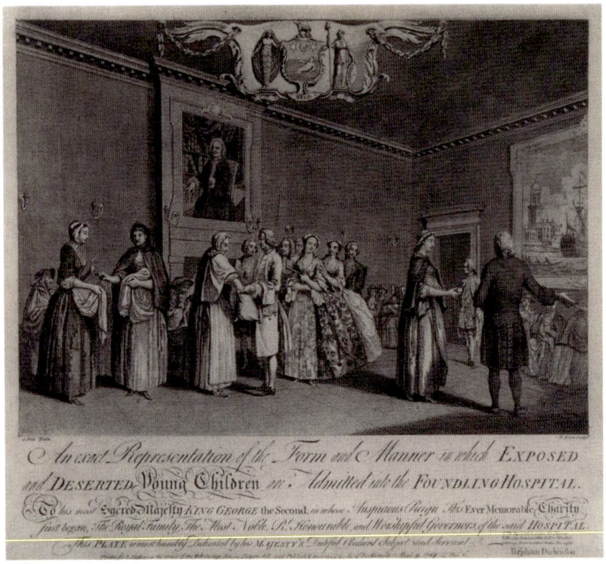

86 Nathaniel Parr after Samuel Wale, *An Exact Representation of the Form and Manner in which Exposed and Deserted Young Children are admitted to the Foundling Hospital*, 1749, etching, 309 x 355 mm, The Foundling Museum, London

to his will: 'To the Governors and Guardians of the Hospital for Poor Children his picture over the chimney in the great parlor at Battersea'.[26] Emerson died in July 1746, also leaving an impressive £12,000 to the Hospital.[27] Highmore's portrait was then prominently displayed in the Foundling Hospital's admissions room (fig. 86) and therefore presided over the desperate scenes played out there, as infants were either accepted or rejected by the Hospital.

However, the encouragement of native artists and the promotion of native art could not exist in isolation from the Hospital's raison d'être, that is, the preservation of babies at risk of abandonment (rather than orphaned children) for the most part presumed to be 'low born' and illegitimate.

In *Painting for Money*, David Solkin sets out the case for the history paintings as a twofold act of benevolence, first as a donation to the Hospital in their own right and secondly, in the feelings of benevolence that they would in turn stimulate in others, via the selecting and effective depiction of relevant subjects.[28] In his *Essays, moral, religious, and miscellaneous* Highmore considered, in relation to 'benevolence',

> the tenderness for children, not only in parents, but in strangers and though that of the former should be distinguished by the term *instinct*, it is not therefore the less natural; for it is supposed, that benevolence is implanted in us by the God of nature, as a principle of action. Hence the pain we feel, on the mere relation of the sufferings of others, who have no connection with us, who are utterly unknown to us, in past ages and distant countries, and the ardent wishes to relieve, even where it is not in our power; the detestation of cruelty, which we properly call *inhumanity*, and the approbation of kind and beneficent actions.[29]

If we consider Highmore's actions when self-consciously combining the role of the painter with the citizen, the desire 'to relieve, even where it is not in our power' found some expression in his approach to the histories of Pamela and Clarissa, while his support of Teresia Constantia Phillips reveals that when he had the power to relieve distress he chose to use it and to great effect. The reference to the 'tenderness' or compassion felt towards children by strangers clearly and directly relates to the Foundling Hospital.

But, regarding history painting, the crucial phrase is 'the pain we feel, on the mere relation of the sufferings of others': in this situation 'relation', or communication rather than proximity, could take place through verbal or visual means.[30] Western art was, after all, steeped in the communication of another's suffering by means of visual re-enactment – in its most extreme and visceral form the martyrdom of saints and Christ's Passion. Here Highmore calls to mind the line of reasoning in George Turnbull's *A Treatise on Ancient Painting* (1740) concerning 'the Designing Arts':

> Whatever touches our publick Sense, and calls into Action our generous, tender, and kind Affections, is that which most agreeably detains our Mind, and employs it. Representations of such Subjects, so soon as they are set to our View, immediately attract us, working upon us in the most pleasing, because in the most humane and social Manner.[31]

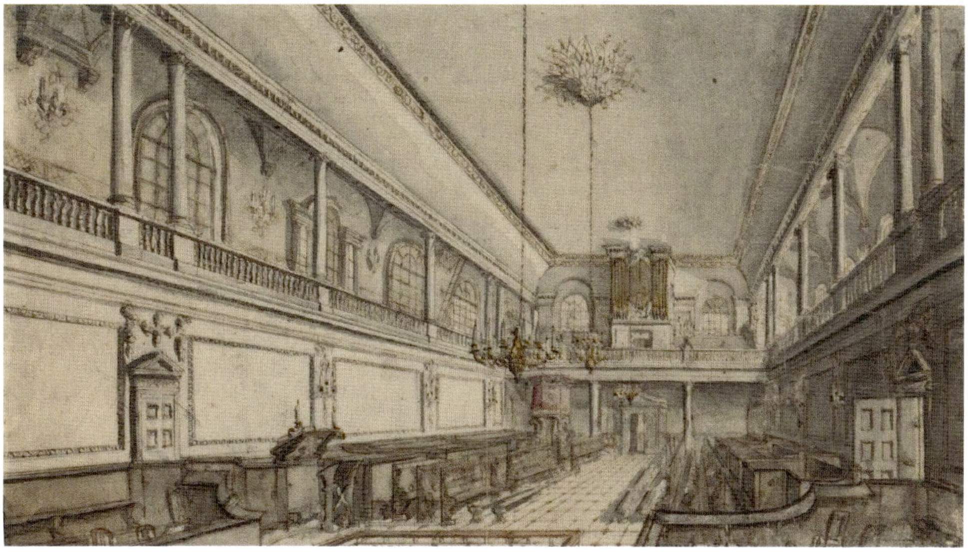

87 Attributed to Theodore Jacobsen, *The chapel of the Foundling Hospital, London*, date not known, watercolour, pen and brown ink over graphite on paper, 187 x 335 mm, Yale Center for British Art, Paul Mellon Collection.

George Frideric Handel (1685–1759) directed a fundraising concert in the unfinished chapel on 27 May 1749, which included the anthem *Blessed are they that considereth the poor*, known as the Foundling Hospital Anthem. Handel, a governor from 1750, then conducted annual performances of his oratorio *Messiah* there until the year of his death. On the demolition of the Hospital, the organ case, pulpit and font were moved to St Andrew's Church, Holborn Circus, along with the remains of Thomas Coram, who had been buried beneath the chapel's altar.

Theodore Jacobsen is listed among Turnbull's subscribers and, although the inclusion of this volume in a connoisseur's library does not confirm direct influence on the design of the Hospital, nonetheless it does suggest that the Hospital's architect was aware of such theories when he was developing his plans for the building (fig. 87). This and the fact that in 1746 Jacobsen had been nominated, along with Hogarth, George Frederick Zincke (1694–1767) and John Michael Rysbrack (1694–1770), as the core members of the annual 'Art Committee', charged with co-ordinating the fine art donations and their display, lead to the assumption that Jacobsen had had a key role in the setting up of the contemporary art programme.[32] Certainly if Jacobsen and his fellow committee members were interested in the effect, as well as existence and location, of the fine art at the Hospital, so too were the artist donors.

In fact a form of 'history painting' in miniature had already been used to represent and promote the Hospital. As the Foundling Hospital project was turning from a theory into a reality, the authorities required a fundraising tool for the purposes of encouraging donations and subscriptions. Perhaps with Hogarth's encouragement, it was decided that the dangers that threatened all infants at risk of abandonment and future foundlings – dangers which included infanticide – could be more directly and therefore more powerfully relayed through graphic illustration. In eighteenth-century Britain images of contemporary abandonment, much less child murder, were extremely rare. Sadly, London newspapers provided evidence of both. The *Universal Spectator and Weekly Journal* of 21 March 1730, under the section 'Diseases and Casualties this Week', reported 'One (a Male Infant) murder'd, in the Church-yard at St Botolph's without Bishopsgate', while in June 1731 the front page of *The Daily Advertiser* informed its readers of a 'murder'd Infant' found 'near the Half-Mile-House' in Dublin, 'which had five or six Stabs of a small Sword in the Head'.[33]

Hogarth's resulting design (fig. 88) of 1738 was engraved by François Morellon La Cave (fl. 1726–66) and

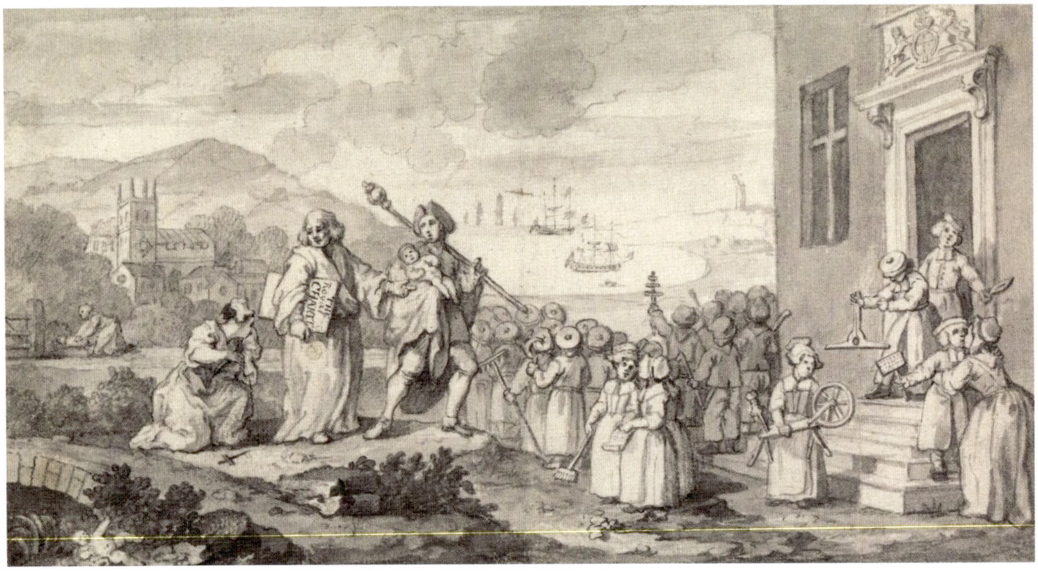

88 William Hogarth, Study for *The Foundlings*, c.1739, pen and ink with grey wash on paper, 111 x 213 mm, Yale Center for British Art, Paul Mellon Collection

published in 1739. The narrative and details within the design were no doubt discussed in advance by those involved in the project, including Coram, and then sanctioned by them. Hogarth's design was therefore the official image circulated to donors and potential donors, and so offers an early representation of the context and purpose of the institution.

The centre of the design is dominated by the figure of the Hospital's beadle, an officer responsible for security, who, along with Coram himself, standing to the left, effectively and symbolically acts as the device separating the rescued foundlings to the right from the acts of abandonment and attempted new-born child murder occurring to the left. Aside from Coram and the beadle, the most prominent figure is the kneeling, weeping woman who has been interrupted in her intention to murder, with the dagger lying in front of her, the small child that the beadle holds. Behind this woman, another is in the process of abandoning an infant by the path, while in the foreground (bottom left) a vulnerable naked child lies by the river. Hogarth offers enough for the viewer to imagine what has just happened and therefore, through the existence of the Foundling Hospital, what horrors have and, in the future, will be avoided. It is surely no coincidence that the window bars of the Hospital are formed into a cross, indicating where Christian charity can be found. What is emphatically clear is the role of the Foundling Hospital as the 'saviour' of these children.

On one level, then, the four history paintings and the stories they revealed were designed, like the subscription roll headpiece, to assist in stirring up feelings of humanity and converting them into acts of benevolence or generosity – particularly financial generosity. How successful the history paintings were in practice is impossible to quantify and it is certainly difficult to imagine a more compelling argument for support than the little foundlings themselves in their brown and red uniforms. At the very least, the paintings were part of a carefully constructed environment, which, on the one hand, provided an appropriate space for entertaining donors and potential donors and, on the other, reflected the benevolent principles of the institution and its governors through the dignified representation of the context, core purpose and beneficiaries of the charity.

'LIFT UP HER VOICE, AND WEPT'

Highmore's subject for his Court Room painting, *Hagar and Ishmael*, comes from the Book of Genesis. Abraham, the first of the Hebrew patriarchs, and his wife Sarah are old and childless. Sarah encourages Abraham to take their Egyptian servant Hagar as a concubine, so that she can conceive a child, Ishmael. Despite her advanced age, Sarah later gives birth to Isaac, the father of the Jewish nation, and instructs Abraham to send Ishmael and Hagar away. Hagar and Ishmael wander through the desert, until the water that Abraham has given them runs out. Hagar places her dying son under a shrub and then moves away from him, 'for she said, Let me not see the death of the child. And she sat over against him, and lift up her voice, and wept.'[34] An angel appears saying, 'What aileth thee, Hagar? fear not; for God hath heard the voice of the lad'.[35] A spring appears, and mother and child are saved.

European artists working in the Western tradition, from the Renaissance onwards, focused on three main episodes from the Hagar story. The first in the sequence is the introduction of Hagar to Abraham by his wife Sarah; the second is the casting out of Hagar and Ishmael; and the last is the scene in the desert. In the first and second, Abraham is present in the composition, reminding us of the dominant partner in the sexual relationship which lies at the story's heart and, more importantly, his role in rejecting and endangering the lives of the woman and their child.[36] Potentially all three narratives have equal relevance to the modern foundling, yet it is the scene in the desert that Highmore and his colleagues deemed most appropriate to the image, purpose and activity of the London Foundling Hospital. It focused on mother and child and visualized an external intervention – divinely inspired as represented by the angel – that delivers both from destruction and death.

Within Highmore's composition (fig. 89) the three figures of Hagar, Ishmael and angel have formed a triangle, with the angel above and Hagar and Ishmael forming the base. The 'triangular' format inevitably creates a space at the centre of the canvas, which is exaggerated if the three figures are pulled to the front of the picture plane. This basic composition is not in itself an innovative response to this narrative: in fact, in the context of Italian and French art, it had become a convention by the seventeenth century.[37] In terms of both composition and style, Highmore consciously placed himself within this Western tradition of history painting. Yet, having chosen this specific composition, Highmore further refined it by depicting a very precise moment from the biblical story, in the full knowledge, it will be argued, of its potential effect upon the Hospital governors and visitors.

Highmore has positioned the angel to the left of top centre and therefore in the same half of the painting as Ishmael, leaving Hagar alone to the right. The composition therefore creates a separation between the lead characters, but most particularly and significantly between the mother and child, Hagar and Ishmael. In the biblical account, Hagar had consciously moved away from her dying son 'as it were a bolt's distance' and turned away from or 'against' him so as not to witness his death. No matter how understandable her reaction might be, rather than holding and comforting her son she is described as having abandoned him. In the context of the Foundling Hospital, this distinction was important and, echoing it, Highmore has shown Hagar kneeling with her body facing away from Ishmael's lifeless form. The artist creates, in effect, the reverse of the Virgin Mary cradling her dead son – a dismantled *Pietà*. Though Hagar becomes aware of the angel's presence and is shown turning towards him, her face continues to show the emotions from the scene previous to this one. Rather than the comfort, or perhaps joy, that we can expect her to feel in a moment from now, Hagar's expression is closer to extreme distress and even fear. Highmore has therefore chosen to represent a moment *between* despair and deliverance. This distinction is crucial, as there are in fact two narratives suggested here. And, regarding the painting's destination, one is dominant over the other.

The first is the actual biblical story, where, after their hardship and misfortune, both the mother and child survive and are reunited. The second is the contemporary story of a woman who is forced through circumstance to leave her child to the care of the Hospital. In regard to the first, this is a narrative representing divine intervention and deliverance that, as stated, forms part of the Western pictorial tradition. However, it can be argued that this particular narrative was neither appropriate nor was required within a refuge for foundlings. Such an interpretation would infer that the Hospital's role was a temporary one, and that the mother and child would be reunited if or when circumstances improved. This argument is certainly supported by the presence of thousands of 'tokens' in the Hospital's archive. These are usually small items made of textile, metal or paper that were left with the infant by the (presumed) mother as a distinguishing marker. The Hospital's documentation of every child on admittance and the accompanying token allowed for identification and therefore the potential for reclamation.

Yet, by 1746, while Highmore was considering his approach to the Hagar story, the Hospital had been receiving children in their temporary buildings at Hatton Garden for over four years and the governors would have been aware that, in practice, very few children were reclaimed. For example, of the 228 children accepted by the Hospital between 1741 and 1745, 118 died within two years and only one was recorded as having been reclaimed.[38] This was in large part due to the Hospital's requirement for reimbursement of expenses on reclamation.[39] It should also be noted that a significant number of the infants were left without tokens.[40]

These facts alone hint at the complexity of the erased histories of the 'abandoned' and the 'abandoner'. This brings us back to the second – and very modern – story reflected in Highmore's painting. Rather than a temporary refuge, the Hospital, as stated in its official title, existed for the 'maintenance' and 'education' of 'exposed and deserted young children'. Further, one of the key stated aims of the Hospital, repeated several times in the petition for establishment presented to King George II in 1737, was the production of honest, useful citizens – surely something they could not guarantee if, in reality, the infants were routinely returned to their mothers.[41] If the angel's action signals the intervention of the Hospital to relieve the suffering of both parent and child, then Highmore registers its role in this 'unnatural' but necessary (and voluntary) separation of mothers from their children through the yellow light that originates, halo-like, around the angel's head and then proceeds down through the centre of the canvas in a jagged motion, effectively severing the canvas in two. It should be stressed that the Hospital's presumed insurance was that the babies were being left with the consent of their mothers. Having been separated from the child, the woman turns back and up to look at the angel, her face betraying fear and anxiety rather than relief and joy. Highmore's depiction of this 'abandoning' mother is dignified and even empathetic, in so far as her suffering is evident. But for this modern Hagar, the relationship with her child will indeed end here.

'A CONJOINT AGREEMENT'

As previously discussed, on one level, the four history paintings and the individual narratives they revealed were designed to assist in creating and then converting feelings of humanity into acts of benevolence. The subjects of the four history paintings are Highmore's *Hagar and Ishmael* (fig. 89); *Little Children brought unto Christ* by Wills (fig. 90); *Moses found in the Bulrushes* by Hayman (fig. 91); and *Moses coming before Pharaoh's Daughter* by Hogarth (fig. 92). The paintings offer a variety of scenarios that resonated with the presumed background and context of the foundling children.[42] For example, Hagar, the servant and concubine of Abraham, would have been recognized as both a victim and as a 'fallen' woman. She is cast out by Abraham along with their son Ishmael, who is the physical evidence of the sexual relationship between Hagar and her 'master'.[43] To a modern British audience this figure and her circumstances could represent the vulnerability of unmarried females in domestic service – the scenario of Samuel Richardson's *Pamela*. In contrast Moses's mother is not a fallen woman, nor is her child illegitimate. She hides Moses to prevent his murder on

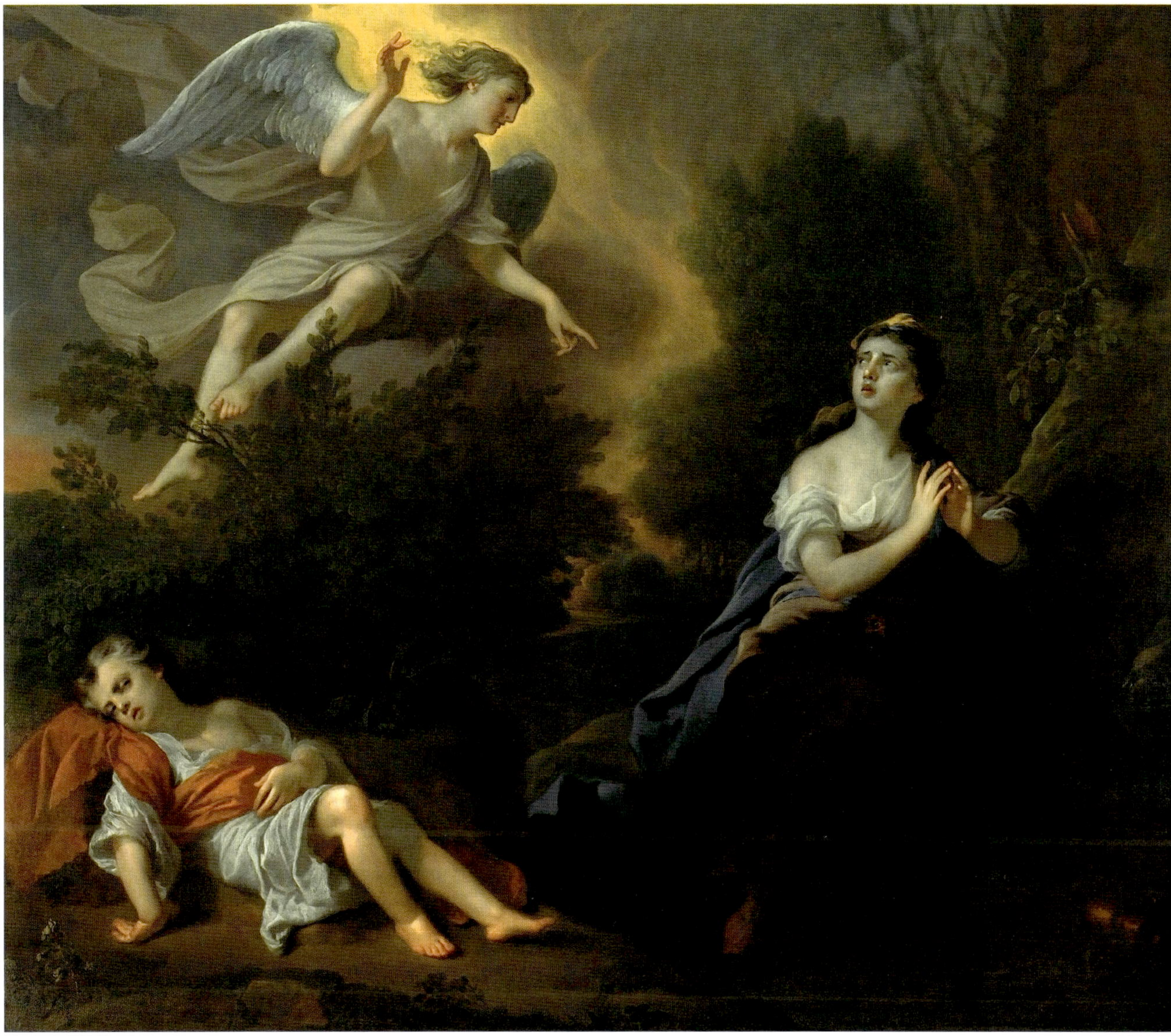

89 Joseph Highmore, *Hagar and Ishmael*, 1746, oil on canvas, 173 x 193 cm, The Foundling Museum, London

the orders of Pharaoh and then contrives to have him discovered by Pharaoh's daughter in order to save his life. In fact, in the biblical narrative, through the guile of her daughter, she is given the role of wet nurse to her own son. This biblical scenario might acknowledge that some of the modern infants left at the Hospital, rather than being illegitimate or 'unwanted', were from loving families who, through extreme circumstances, were forced into this desperate act in the hope of offering the infant a chance of survival or a better life. The scheme therefore provided useful models for the sympathetic representation of the foundlings' natural mothers.

The paintings also offer clear demonstrations of compassionate and charitable behaviour in action and therefore served as powerful models for the potential donor. In Highmore's painting, Ishmael, abandoned and dying, is rescued through the intervention of God by means of an angel: the Hayman and Hogarth

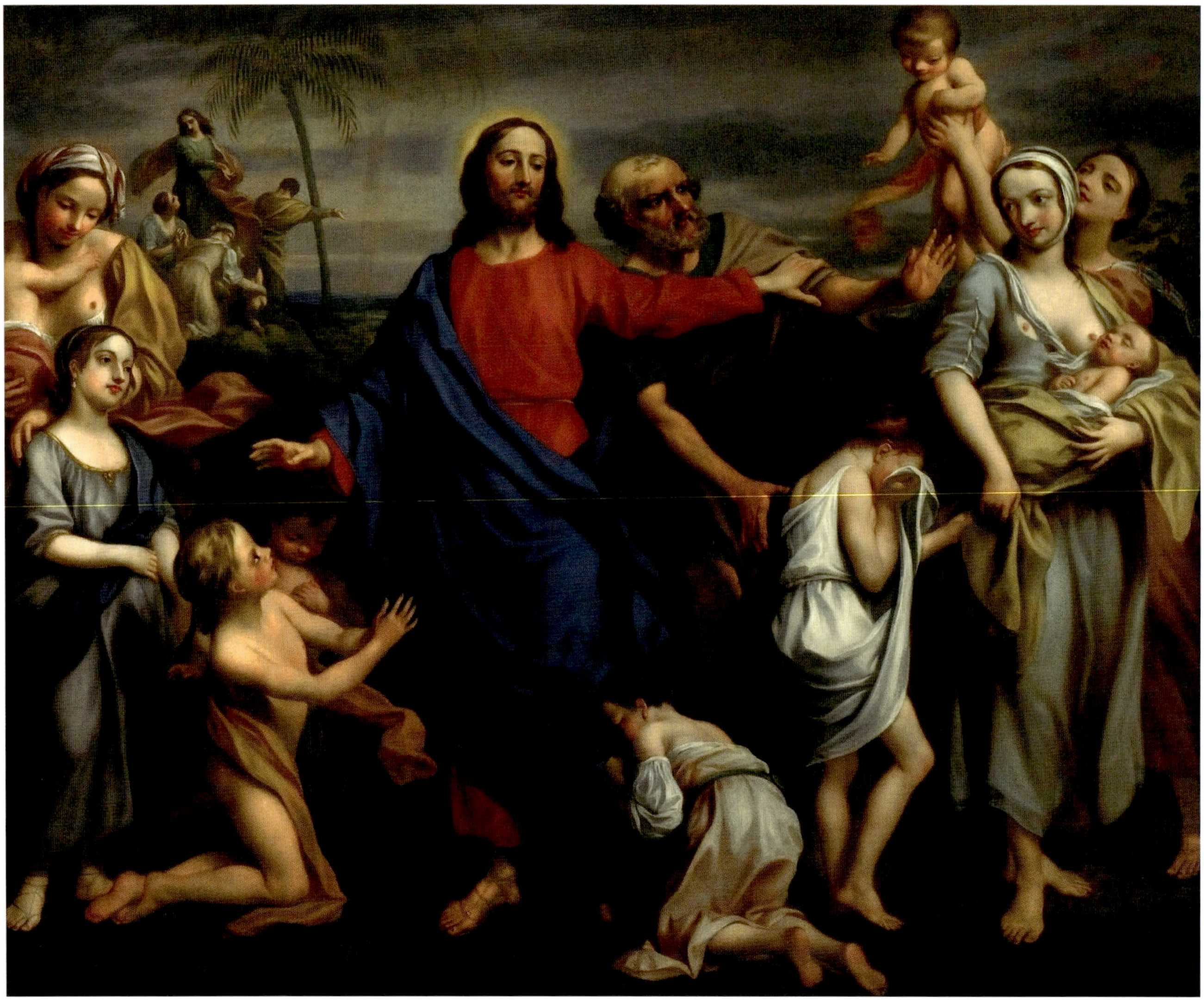

90 James Wills, *Little Children brought unto Christ*, 1746, oil on canvas, 172.7 x 209 cm, The Foundling Museum, London

James Wills was a member of Hogarth's St Martin's Lane Academy (formed in 1735) and had studied in Italy. He was later ordained as a priest.

paintings depict, respectively, the rescue and then adoption of Moses by Pharaoh's daughter, and, in Wills's canvas, Jesus instructs his disciples to 'Suffer the little children to come unto me, and forbid them not: for of such is the kingdom of God'.[44] The four artists have distanced the main figures from recognizable inhabitants of the Near East by representing them as Western, as opposed to ancient Egyptian or Jewish. Crucially both children, Ishmael and Moses, are blond with very pale skin. Although it was an accepted convention within European art selectively to 'westernize' biblical figures, in this setting such a treatment signals the existence of a parallel story firmly located within modern Britain.

Further, if viewed as an independent image, each canvas represents a child who has been saved from death in order to fulfil his destiny. Ishmael is destined to found the 'Arab' nation and Moses leads his people

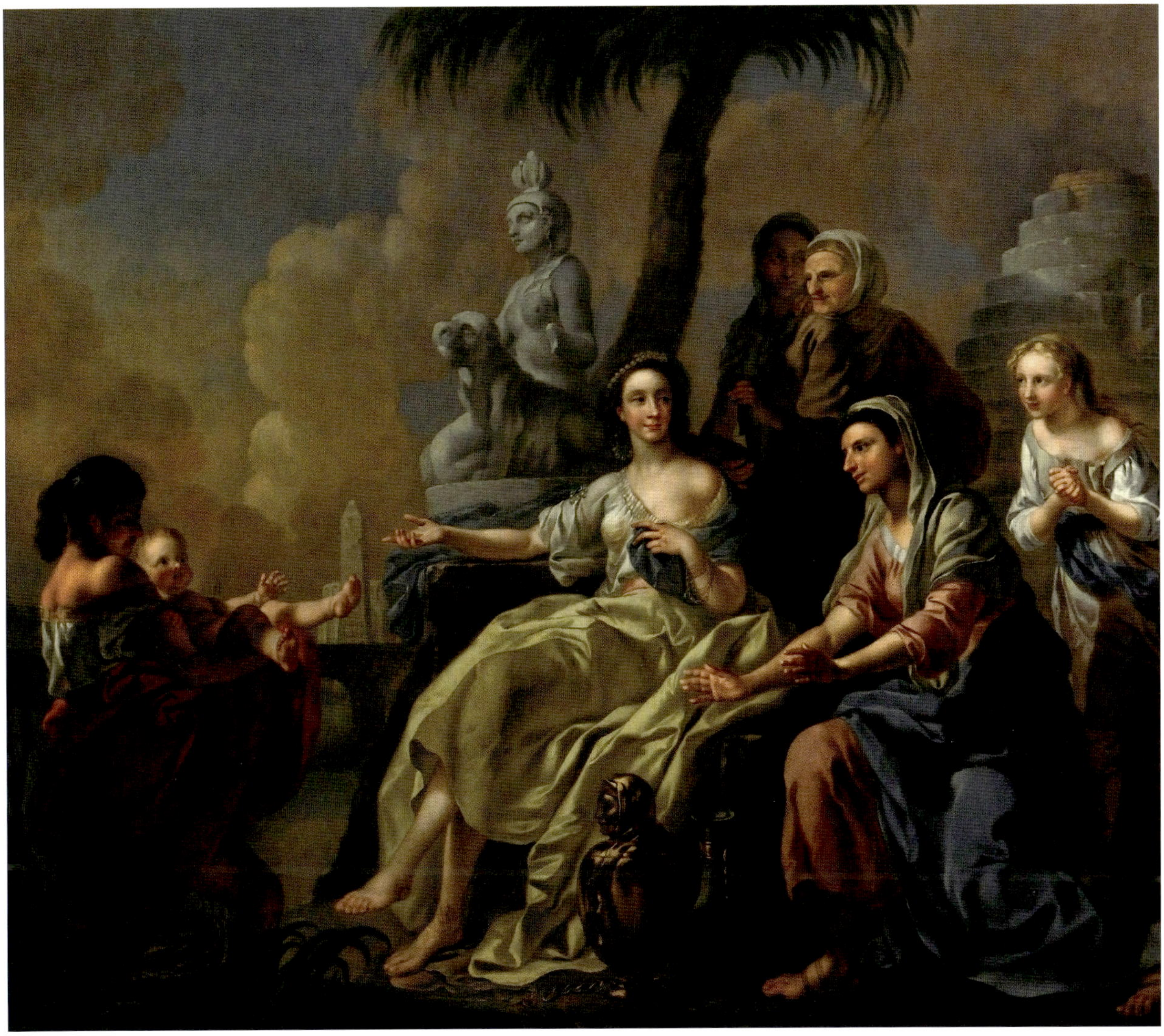

91 Francis Hayman, *Moses found in the Bulrushes*, 1746, oil on canvas, 172.7 x 208 cm, The Foundling Museum, London

out of slavery to the Promised Land. The presence of the mature Jesus of Nazareth within the iconography of a Foundling Hospital may have reminded the viewer of the fraught and humble circumstances of Jesus's own birth and infancy and particularly the violent story of the Massacre of the Innocents. Even God, in the form of His son, was once a vulnerable baby, dependent on the behaviour of the adults around him for his safety. This helpless child is rescued and, for Christians, matures into the ultimate role model. To a lesser degree, the children supported through the Foundling Hospital will achieve a suitable and useful destiny, useful, that is, to society and the British nation, as the petition to the king in council of 1737 had made clear.[45] As Matthew Henry noted in 1725, with reference to Ishmael's rescue, 'it should engage our Care and Pains about Children and young People, to consider, that we know not what God has designed 'em for, nor what great use Providence may make of them'.[46]

Hitherto it had been presumed that the paintings were linked simply by the fact that they each depicted a biblical narrative connected to children,

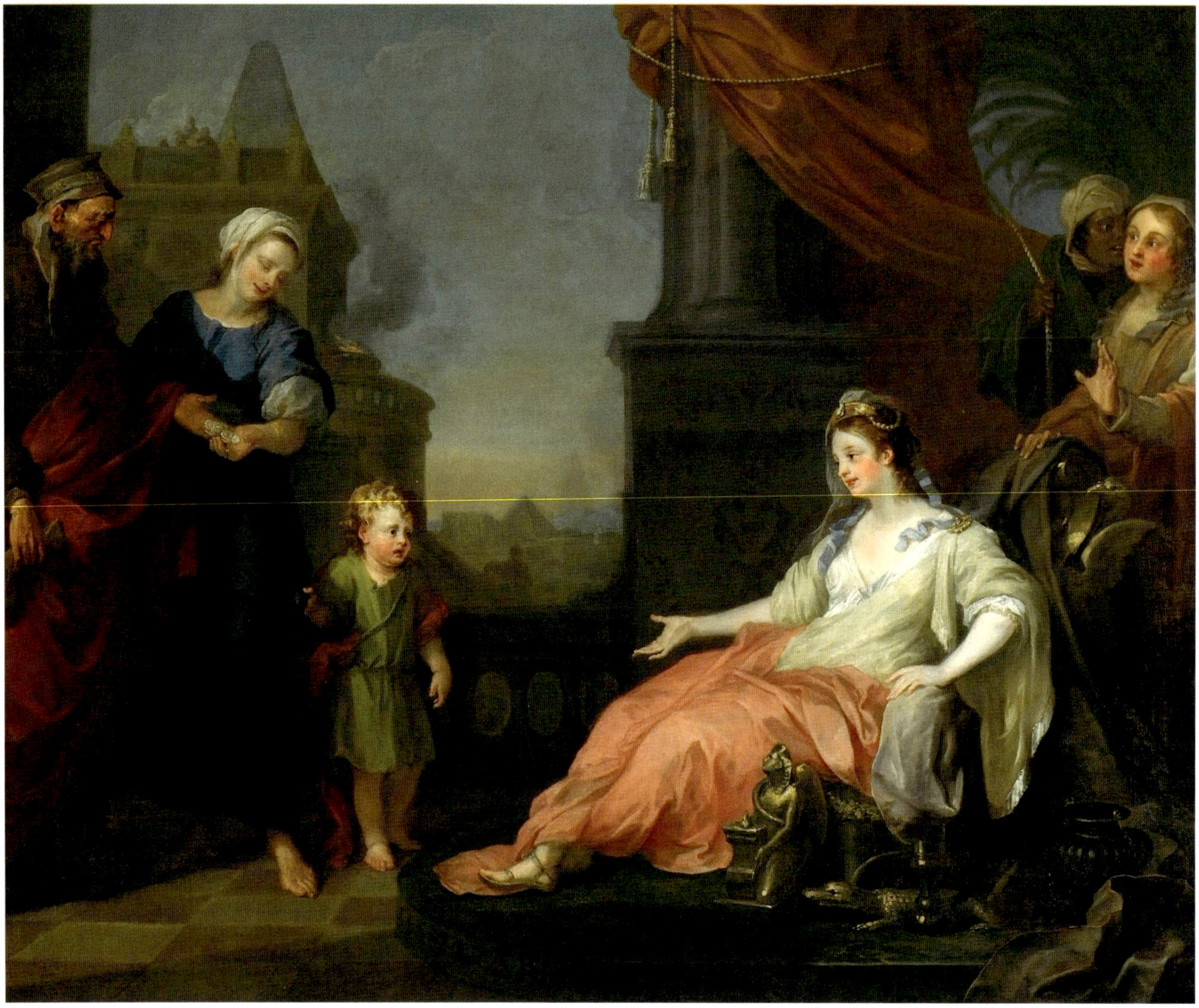

92 William Hogarth, *Moses coming before Pharaoh's Daughter*, 1746, oil on canvas, 172.7 x 208 cm, The Foundling Museum, London

as outlined above.[47] Further, the attention and focus given by scholars of eighteenth-century British art to Hogarth's *Moses* has effectively isolated his painting from its companions.[48] As a result, the four paintings continued to be judged as essentially independent images. Thus any potential that they might reveal a more sophisticated collective approach when analysed together has been overlooked. However, John Brownlow, the first historian of the Hospital, writing in the mid nineteenth century, stated that the history painting scheme within the Court Room was a 'conjoint agreement' between the four artists.[49] Brownlow's statement introduces the possibility that the four artists worked closely together to produce four images that, if read as a sequence, provided a unified and dominant narrative.

The key is the arrangement of the paintings within the Court Room. The current Court Room in the Foundling Museum is a reconstruction, but the photographs of the room in the original Foundling

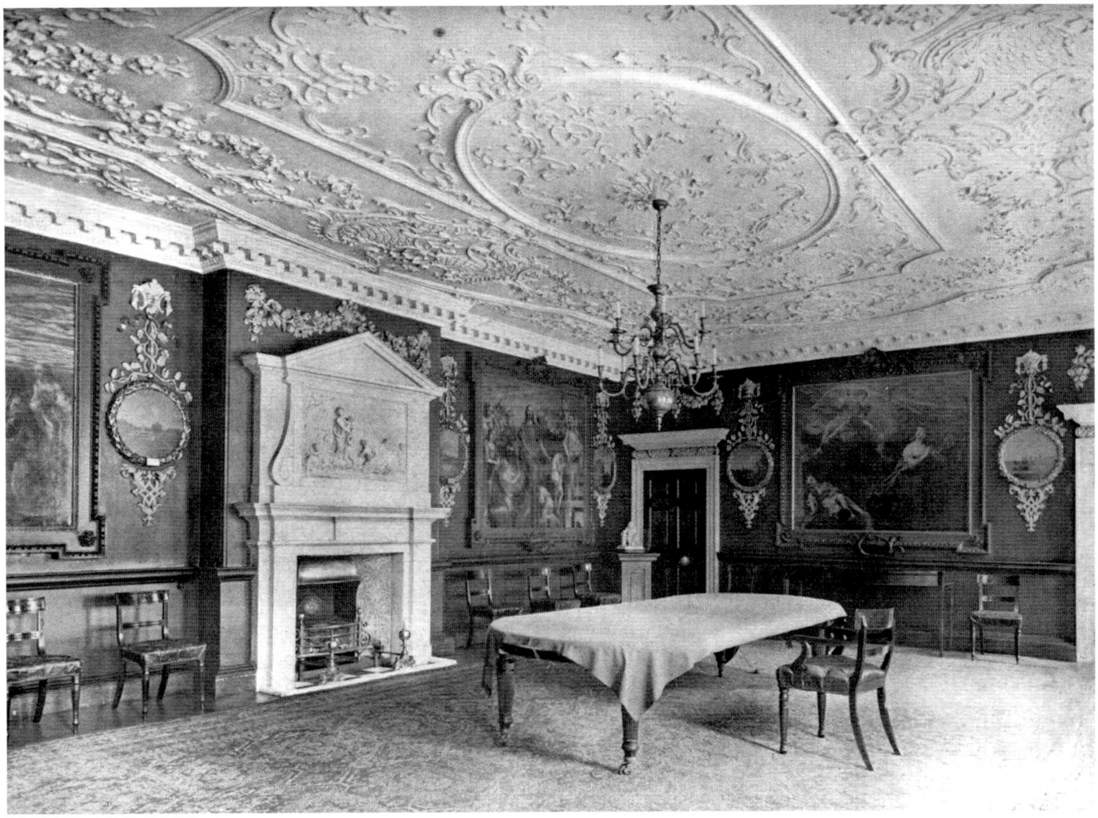

93 The Governors' Court Room in the Foundling Hospital, photographed before 1926

Hospital building (fig. 93) taken just prior to its sale in 1926 and demolition make clear that the paintings were in their current sequence in the 1920s and presumably had been so since their donation. The early commentaries of the Court Room's contents, which are barely more than lists, offer no concrete challenge to this presumption. The first official description of the Hospital, *An Account of the Hospital for the Maintenance and Education of Exposed and Deserted Young Children*, dated 1749, lists them as 1) Hayman 2) Hogarth 3) Highmore 4) Wills, whereas, in 1755, Rouquet lists them as 1) Hayman 2) Hogarth 3) Wills 4) Highmore.[50] Both observers appear to pair them 'correctly' on either side of Rysbrack's marble overmantle (to the left Hayman/Hogarth and the right Wills/Highmore), but neither offers confirmation as to precise location and therefore sequence. If we return to the current hang within the reconstructed Court Room, its authenticity becomes more likely if a narrative linking the four individual subjects can be proposed.

The current hang still presents two ways of approaching the sequence. But by replaying the subjects from Hogarth to Highmore a new problem arises. For example, Moses returns as a child to Pharaoh's daughter in Hogarth's painting, and then would be found by her as an infant in the adjoining painting by Hayman. The relationship between the Hogarth and Hayman paintings is only resolved if the sequence is reversed. Does this suggest an overarching narrative from Highmore through Wills and Hayman to Hogarth?

In Highmore's canvas, an abandoned child is rescued through a timely intervention; in the Wills canvas, children are encouraged to approach their

Saviour, rather than being prevented from doing so; in Hayman's painting, the infant's new patron or foster parent delivers him for a temporary period only to a wet nurse, and, finally, in the Hogarth, the grown child returns to the care of his patron/foster parent. Therefore, the scheme appears to symbolize the progress or 'processing' of the modern foundling child from 1) abandonment as a baby, via 2) the initial reception at the Hospital and then 3) sending out to be wet-nursed in the country, to 4) the return and full admission to the Hospital at the age of about three.[51] This reading is then shaped by the movement from an actual mother, Hagar, to an adoptive mother, Pharaoh's daughter: from the humble modern 'birth mother' to the protecting, authoritative 'institutional mother', the Hospital. In theory both offer different but equally valid symbols of mothering and nurturing, but, when located within the Foundling Hospital, it is the latter, in the face of the birth mother's inability to protect and preserve her offspring, which is demonstrably the more successful. It is the Hospital therefore that comes to represent parental protection and care, not the child's natural parent. The natural mothers are unimportant here, or at least secondary: the biblical narrative tells us that it is Ishmael's cries that are heard by God, not Hagar's; the children, not their mothers, are bidden to come to Jesus; Moses's biological mother is given an important but secondary role as a wet nurse and is then paid off and dismissed.

To echo this, at the beginning of the sequence Highmore has depicted a space at the centre of the canvas to establish the separation between the figures of Hagar and Ishmael, mother and child, and then emphasized it through the jagged light that is splitting the canvas in two. Scholars have highlighted the significance of the narrow central space between Moses and Pharaoh's daughter within Hogarth's painting, but such spatial symbolism is evident in all four canvases and in turn supports the idea of a connecting narrative.[52] In the compositions of Hayman, Hogarth and Wills, the figures are gathered and grouped, not isolated, and in each case the separation of the children or child from their adult protector is in the process of being broken down. In Wills's canvas, located immediately to the left of Highmore's, the children are no longer discouraged from approaching the central figure of Jesus and are shown either tentatively touching the hem of his clothing or still in tears at St Peter's reprimand. In Hayman's canvas, the recently discovered infant Moses is being carried to the outstretched arms of his wet nurse/natural mother with his adoptive mother looking contentedly on. In the case of Hogarth's painting, the culmination of the series, the unsettling space first opened up by Highmore's *Hagar and Ishmael* is about to be closed by the child Moses, who will soon reach up to take the already extended hand of Pharaoh's daughter. In its composition, therefore, Highmore's canvas creates a visual contrast to the relative balance and order of the other three and, further, depicts an uneasy, unnatural breach that is finally 'repaired' within Hogarth's *Moses*.

Hogarth had already rehearsed a type of 'episodic' storyline within his earlier subscription roll headpiece. From left to right the three 'groupings' of 1) mothers and infants 2) Coram, baby and beadle and 3) the uniformed foundlings with their spindles and sextants can be read as symbolizing 1) danger/abandonment, 2) rescue/reception and finally 3) maintenance/nurture. Further, the argument presented here is supported by the contemporary descriptions already quoted above. The first official Foundling Hospital description introduces the Court Room history paintings in the following manner: 'the Subjects being Parts of the Sacred History, suitable to the Place for which they were designed'.[53] Add to this Rouquet's specific use of the phrase 'the exposed children' rather than simply 'children' in his statement, 'the subjects are all taken from scripture, and relate to the exposed children',[54] and it becomes clear that, for contemporary viewers at least, the modern foundling's history of despair and hope was a constant and highly visible – if somewhat sanitized – presence through the Court Room's history paintings. The biblical sources assisted in this distancing and then elevation from what was a terrible reality, lending gravitas, pedigree, legitimacy and even spirituality to this modern moral subject.

'THE HEINOUSNESS OF THE CRIME'

The abandoning of children was one part of this terrible reality that the Hospital sought to address. As noted earlier, another was new-born child murder.[55] Separating actual murder, whether premeditated or on the spur of the moment, from the death of a child due to lack of awareness or through want of basic care and assistance was far from straightforward. The terrible case of the dead infant discovered with the multiple stab-wounds to the head, as reported in *The Daily Advertiser* in 1731, seems clear enough (although the gender of the perpetrator less so). Yet the Old Bailey trials for new-born child murder (commonly called 'infanticide'), where the accused were predominantly unmarried females, reveal the difficulty in establishing motivation and intent.[56] On 28 August 1730 Elizabeth Smith, an unmarried servant of St Margaret's, Westminster, was tried for 'the Murther of her Female Bastard Infant, by throwing it into a Vault, by which it was suffocated and strangled'. Elizabeth had clearly attempted to hide her pregnancy, but argued that she had gone to the vault because she had 'a violent looseness' of the bowels and had then unexpectedly given birth, dropping and killing the child in error. In court it was confirmed that there were 'no marks of violence on the body' and, in the opinion of the midwife witness, a sudden unexpected birth was not unusual. However, the key was whether 'the Prisoner made Provision for the Child', in other words, had she purchased clothing in anticipation of keeping rather than murdering the child? As 'one Child's cap' along with other items were found among her belongings, she was acquitted.[57]

Similarly, Elizabeth Turner, another unmarried servant in Clerkenwell, who was tried on 30 June 1734 for the murder of her baby son, had given birth in secret and then attempted to hide the body in a wig box in the cellar of her mistress's house. The smell from the rotting 'mouldy' corpse led to the discovery, but once again, the presence of 'Babby things' among her possessions, on arrival at Newgate prison, was enough to acquit her.[58] Very occasionally convictions did occur.[59] In the case of Elizabeth Ambrook the discovery of baby linen – in this instance believed to have been planted after the fact to assist in her acquittal – was ignored. According to witnesses her new-born boy was found on the roof of a shed, having been (by her own admission) flung from a nearby window. The verdict was guilty and the sentence death by hanging.[60]

Highmore would have been aware of Hogarth's subscription roll design, even before his official involvement with the Foundling Hospital project. Its candour in attempting to visualize the problematic circumstances of the foundling child would have made an impression upon him. Yet, it should be noted, while abandonment is shown actual or attempted new-born child murder in progress is not. Even so Hogarth's image might well have informed Highmore's initial thoughts on his *Hagar and Ishmael* painting. That he made preliminary sketches is recorded by Highmore's grandson, Anthony, in 1814, writing that 'Mr. Highmore gave his picture of Hagar and Ishmael, the first study for which is with several others now in the hands of his grand-daughter, Mrs. Sarah Highmore, at Canterbury'.[61] No studies directly linked to Hagar and Ishmael are currently known, but the small oil 'sketch' known as '*The Angel of Mercy*' (fig. 94) may be such a 'first study' or preliminary idea for Highmore's Foundling Hospital gift. However, as we shall see, by the very nature of its imagery and narrative it is more likely to be a separate painting that emerged from Highmore's association with the Foundling Hospital and was worked on in tandem with, or subsequent to, the completion of his history painting.

The scene occurs within a cave or perhaps the ruin of a stone structure that opens out to the left. Within the cave/ruin and dominating the composition are three figures. At the centre is a seated young woman and to the left an angel who, with his back to the viewer, turns towards the woman and holds her right arm, while simultaneously indicating with his left hand through the arched doorway or opening towards the distant silhouette of a building. The third figure, standing to the right, is cloaked and hooded – only the face, one hand and a bare foot are visible – and is in the process of turning away or cowering from the angel and woman.

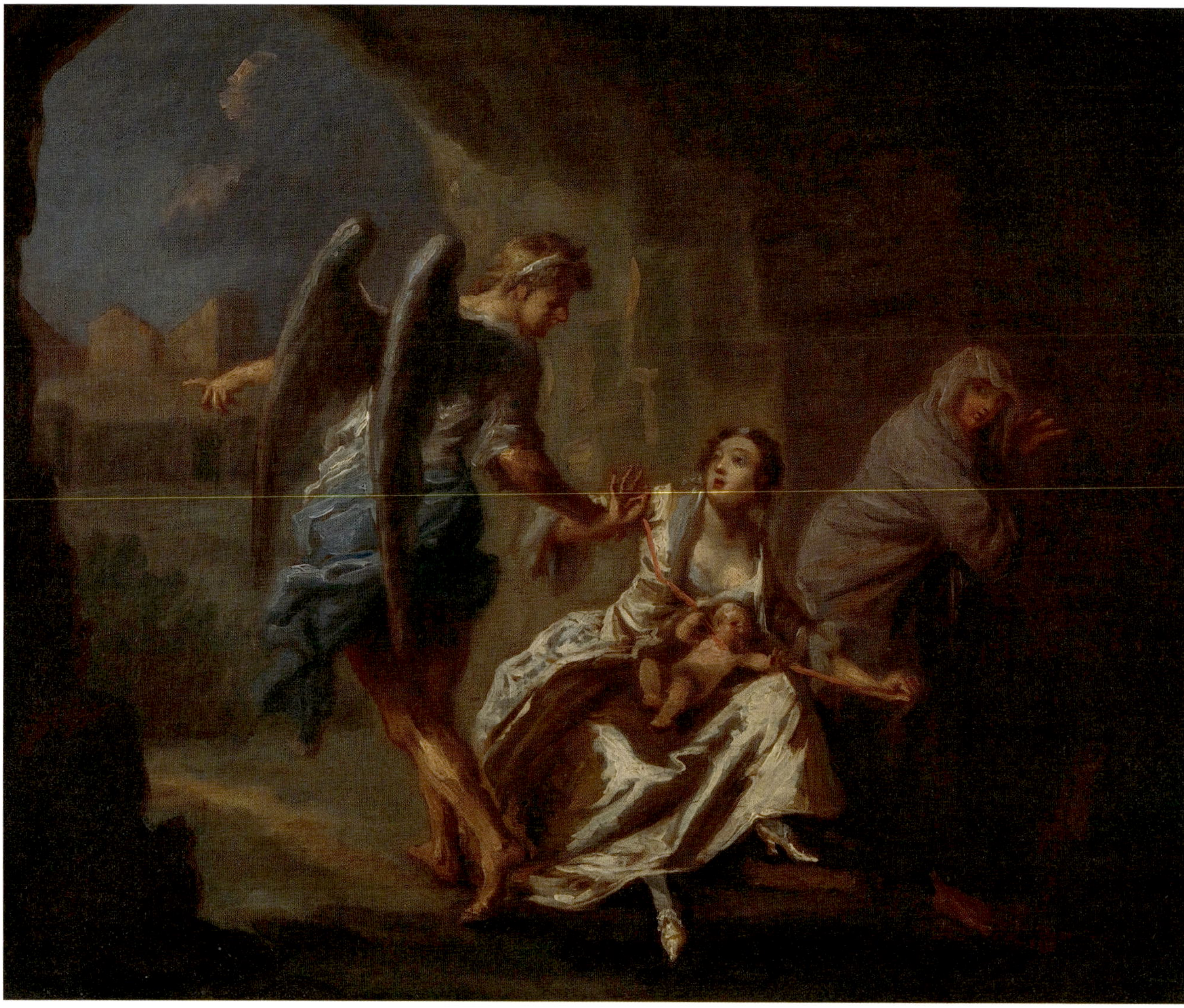

94 Joseph Highmore, *The Angel of Mercy*, c.1746, oil on canvas, 59.7 x 48.3 cm, Yale Center for British Art, Paul Mellon Collection

On closer inspection, the woman is well dressed – the swift 'lightning' highlights across the robe, bodice and underskirt suggest a rich silk – and on her lap is a naked baby. Looking again at the woman's attire, she appears in a state of undress: her robe is loosened, exposing more fully her undergarment and breasts. This may reflect the looser style of clothing worn by pregnant or breast-feeding women. The woman's posture does not correspond with the 'elegance' of her attire, in particular the awkward attitude of her parted legs. She is holding the ends of a coral-pink cord or, more likely, a ribbon in her outstretched hands. It is then evident that the ribbon encircles the child's neck. The woman's disarranged clothing and ungainly stance suggest a corresponding 'derangement' in her mental state.

As contemporary tokens of love, ribbons were popular items left with the infants on admission to the Foundling Hospital (figs. 95 and 96). Of the ten billet books covering the first decade of admissions (1741–51), representing 751 children, in 221 instances ribbons are

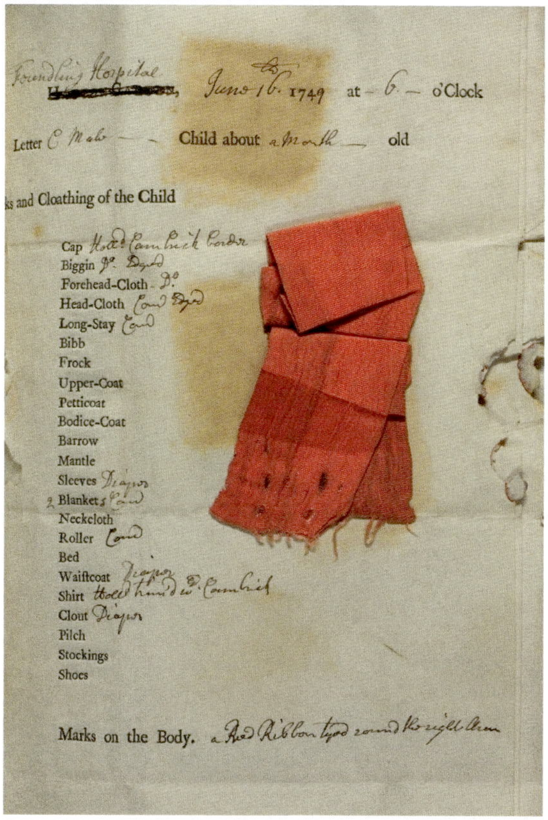

95 A/FH/A/09/01/006 Billet book, male child No.505 with 'a Red Ribbon tyed round the right Arm'

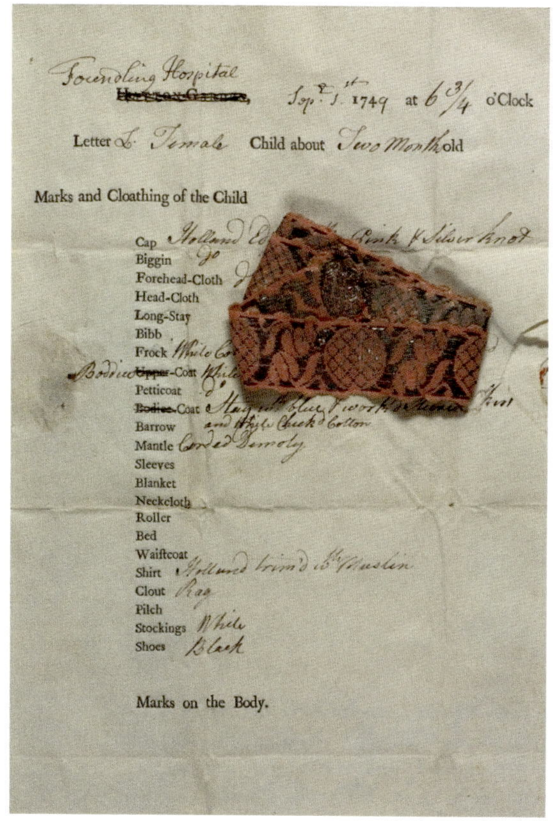

96 A/FH/A/09/01/007 Billet book, female child No.522 with a fine 'Pink & Silver knot' listed with her cap

recorded but no longer present. Coupled with the 47 ribbons which have been recorded and preserved in the archive, this means that well over one third of the infants admitted in this period had ribbons as tokens, a fact that would bring even greater potency to its representation as a weapon of murder.[62] Further, a vast majority of these 268 infants were girls. The top knot and cap ribbon are recognized signifiers of a female child, while ribbons associated with boys appear as cockades (crosses/rosettes), ribbons tied to limbs, or used to attach a token such as a coin.[63] A cap ribbon – in an identical colour to the ribbon or sash present in *The Angel of Mercy* – can be seen in Highmore's portrait *Mrs Sharpe and her Child* (fig. 97). Comparison between the woman in *The Angel of Mercy* and this other new mother – the latter's restrained posture, tentative smile, and the gentleness and pride in which she presents her cherished offspring – confirms the collapse of maternal feeling in the former. Her disordered appearance and splayed legs may also indicate that she has very recently given birth.

Through such means, Highmore establishes that there is a direct relationship between the child and the woman: it is *her* child that she is in the process of killing. The ruined surroundings in which she sits signify her ruin. The traditional representation of the Virgin and Child which Mrs Sharpe and her infant imitate – Highmore included a parrot, a bird associated with the Virgin Mary – has been further subverted by the apparent intimacy and physical closeness of the woman and her infant in *The Angel of Mercy*, which in reality signals danger for one and calamity for both.

As hinted earlier, within Western iconography the established personification of Charity was a suckling

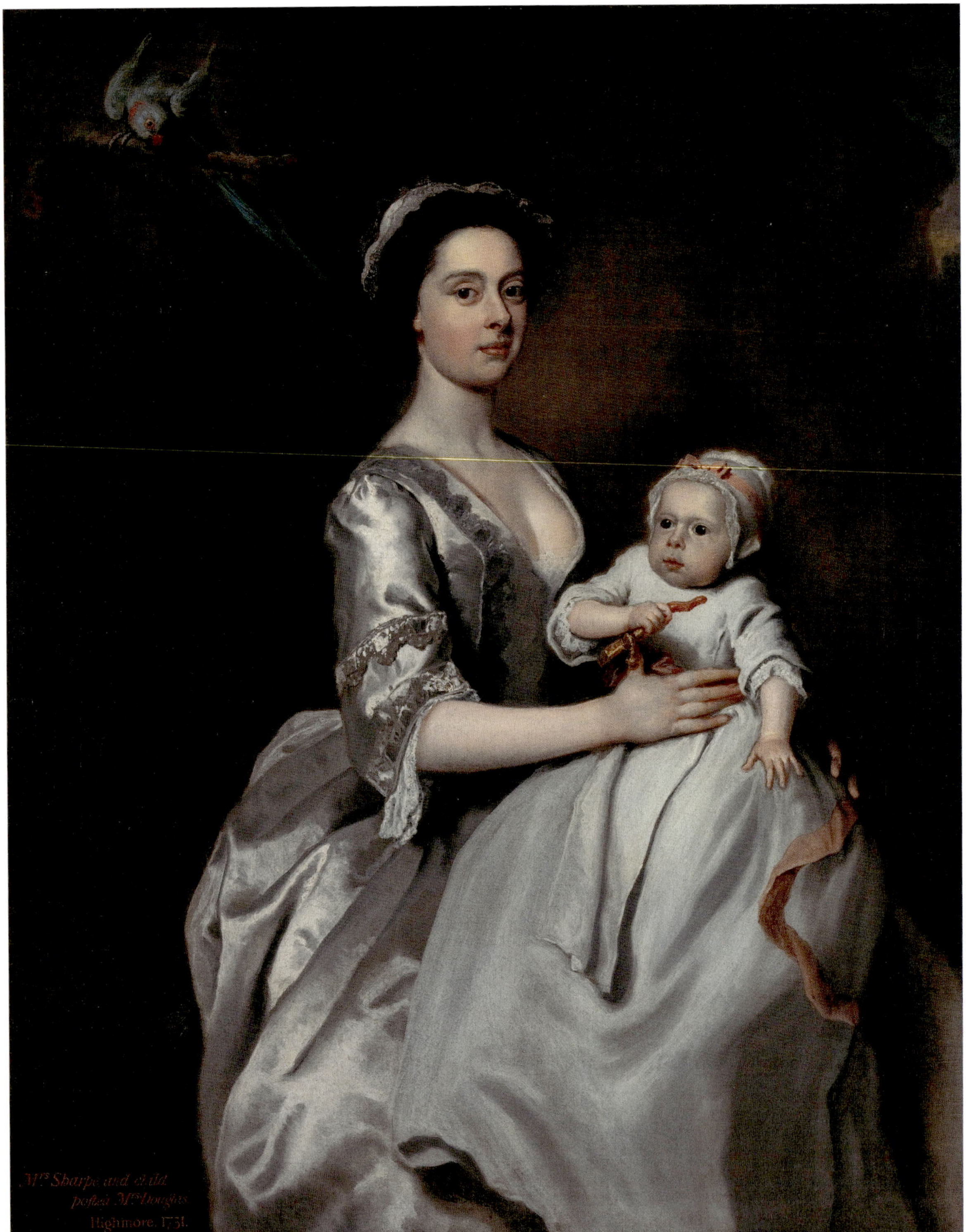

97 Joseph Highmore, *Mrs Sharpe and her Child*, 1731, oil on canvas, 127 x 101.6 cm, Yale Center for British Art, Paul Mellon Collection

and nurturing mother figure, as seen in Rysbrack's overmantle in the Governors' Court Room (fig. 98) and in Highmore's twelfth 'Pamela' scene. In contrast one personification of Cruelty was an infanticidal woman.[64] The former reveals the instinct to protect and nourish the innocent and vulnerable, the latter the urge to misuse a position of control and power, betraying what were seen as correct or natural female impulses. The woman in *The Angel of Mercy* is perhaps a conflation of 'Charity' and 'Cruelty', suggesting that both personae can – or must? – exist within this woman, driven to kill her own child. Within the variety of circumstances that might bring a woman to this resolution, fuelled by an unusual or extreme mental or emotional state, in some instances death might be considered a release, when compared to the imagined life, for both mother and child, should the child live. Occasionally contemporary newspapers offered evidence of such motivation. In Elizabeth Ambrook's case, the flinging of her illegitimate child from a window has all the appearance of an improvised, spur-of-the-moment act, motivated by fear of discovery and the resulting opprobrium of her employer and neighbours. However, the Buckinghamshire mother reported in *The Westminster Journal* in October 1745 to have killed two of her children, and then attempted to kill herself, as a direct result of mounting public hysteria over the advancing Jacobite army – some believed the Highland contingent fed off human flesh – could be viewed, given the terrible rumours, as an act of mercy.[65]

Highmore grappled with the motivation behind new-born child murder in his essay 'On Reputation', in which he considers the maintenance of reputation for men and women in general as a powerful motivation in society. Having contemplated the practice of duelling as the male example, he then states:

> The case of women murdering their illegitimate off-spring is still stronger, inasmuch as very few, if any, of them, have the least doubt of the commonly received notions of religion, or of the heinousness of the crime they are prompted to commit; and it is manifest, that the fear of infamy, or (which is the same thing) a regard for their reputation, is the only motive in many, and the strongest in most, to such crimes, from which the prospect of damnation has not force enough to deter them; so superlatively strong is this principle![66]

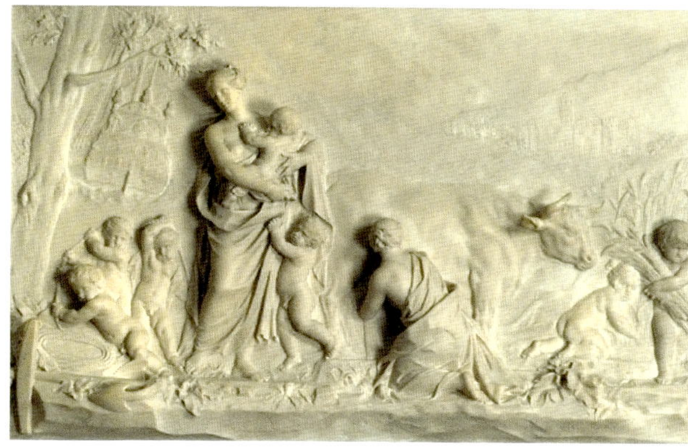

98 John Michael Rysbrack, *Charity* (detail), 1746, marble, 75 x 122 cm, The Foundling Museum, London

Such an assessment appears to disregard the multitude of circumstances that would lead a woman to kill her illegitimate child, although it was an opinion shared by the governors of the Foundling Hospital, as this reference to the purpose of the Hospital (from the General Committee Minutes of 13 December 1739) confirms: '... in order to prevent the frequent murders committed on poor miserable infants by their Parents to hide their shame'.[67]

Yet in the trivializing of societal concepts of 'reputation' – trivial when weighed against murder and damnation, in Highmore's opinion – the critique is as great, if not greater, against the 'society' that encourages such acts, as against the perpetrator herself. Highmore's focus is on the act of murder as a crime against humanity and ultimately God, resulting in wasteful death and eternal damnation, rather than any moral qualm about sex outside of marriage or the child's illegitimacy. With an economy of brush-strokes Highmore creates a look that combines shame, desperation and terror in the woman's blanched face, a detail that hints at an ambivalence towards her plight – on the one hand, a sympathy for the horror of her circumstances, but, more powerful still, an abhorrence

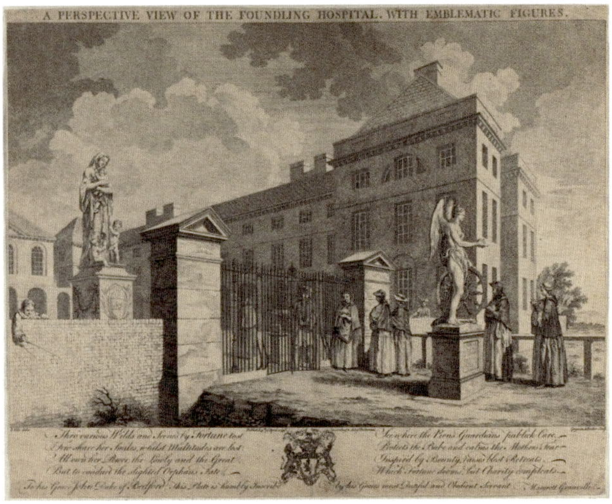

99 Charles Grignion after Samuel Wale, *A Perspective View of the Foundling Hospital with Emblematic Figures*, 1749, etching and line engraving on paper, 350 x 441 mm, Yale Center for British Art, Paul Mellon Collection

of the act she is committing, her abandonment of what he considers Christian values or accepted 'notions of religion' and her want of humanity. Whatever the hostility and rejection that might, or will, result, Highmore might say, surely a child's life is worth the suffering of it?

The taint of illegitimacy and the censure meted out to unmarried mothers were not confined to any single class. When Tom Jones, the most famous foundling after Moses, is discovered in Squire Allworthy's bed, the housekeeper Mrs Deborah Wilkins immediately declares that the 'Hussy its Mother', like all 'such wicked Sluts', should be 'committed to *Bridewel*, and whipt at the Cart's Tail', not knowing that the mother in question was the Squire's unmarried sister Bridget.[68] Fielding's Deborah Wilkins is a caricature of fiction, but the attitude of neighbours and fellow servants, as seen in the Old Bailey infanticide cases, particularly where the unmarried women had hidden their pregnancies, was often unsympathetic, if not aggressively condemning. There is no indication within the composition – for example in the style of her dress – that this woman should be viewed as a prostitute or courtesan (another presumed 'beneficiary' of the Hospital). Highmore is precise enough in his imagery to have removed such ambiguity. The barefooted figure to the right is more beggar than bawd and in all likelihood allegorical. In fact there is a resemblance in the quality of the seated woman's attire, if not the precise style of her dress, to the clothing worn by the emphatically 'middling-sort' wife and mother Mrs Sharpe. Highmore's controversial message appears to be that 'well-born' women, not just the poor, are capable of abandoning, or even murdering their children. Here Highmore seems to be specifically focusing on a woman with an elevated position in society and therefore an associated 'reputation' to maintain.

However, in his *The Angel of Mercy* Highmore offers another path. A significant detail in the composition is the silhouette in the distance (top left) representing the distinctive south view of the Foundling Hospital (compare fig. 99). The central chapel is flanked by the two wings, which are dramatically foreshortened. The forecourt is also seen and, encircling this, the gate and outer wall.[69] The appearance of the Foundling Hospital, like the woman's attire, suggests a date of the mid 1740s. The angel is therefore indicating another future for this woman, one in which, rather than murder her child, she places it in the care of the Hospital. Here then, the Foundling Hospital once more represents the assumed role of saviour and foster parent, as intimated in Hogarth's subscription roll design and later stated in the uniting narrative of the four history paintings of the Governors' Court Room.

Indeed, in *The Angel of Mercy*, Highmore has reinvented, recast and updated the biblical story of Hagar and Ishmael, fusing it with narratives surrounding the modern foundling and the paternalistic principles of the Hospital. As seen in his *Hagar and Ishmael*, the 'angel of mercy' directly intervenes to prevent the death of the child and indicates towards a means of preservation. Yet the arrangement of child, mother and angel has been augmented by the appearance of the figure to the right. Highmore has not committed this figure to a male or female persona and this ambiguity allows for a variety of interpretations. Within the parameters of traditional variations of the Virgin and Child theme, perhaps Highmore is pointedly referring to the Virgin Mary's

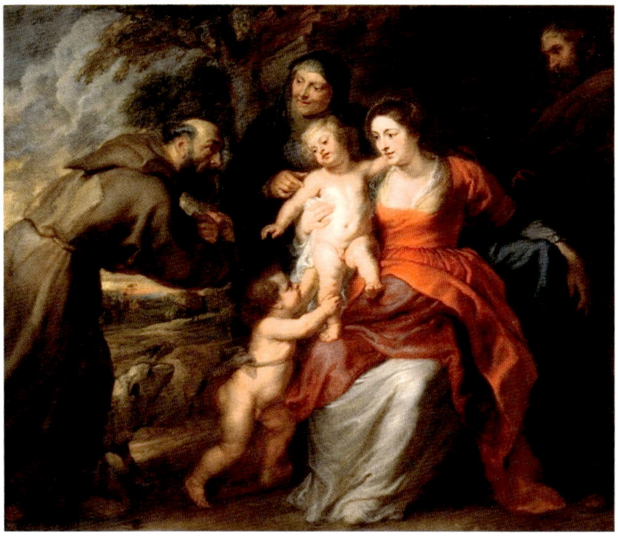

100 Sir Peter Paul Rubens, *The Holy Family with Sts Francis and Anne and the Infant St John the Baptist*, early or mid 1630s, oil on canvas, 176.5 x 209.6 cm, The Metropolitan Museum of Art, New York, Gift of James Henry Smith, 1902

mother, St Anne, often depicted in a full-length black garment and covered head (fig. 100). St Anne is a prime example of a loving mother and grandmother. Such associations emphasize still further the disconnect between the figures of *The Angel of Mercy* and therefore the unnatural collapse of familial and maternal relations: this cowering accomplice to attempted infanticide is the absolute antithesis of St Anne's protecting matriarch.

The shrouded figure may be an allegorical representation of shame, deceit or fraud, as represented in Western pictorial tradition. Further, in its posture as well as attire, the figure appears to mimic Mr B. in Scene 7 of Highmore's 'Pamela' (see fig. 40), a scene charged with male voyeurism and sexual predation. The appearance of similar visual motifs in both compositions – a disguised figure, the dishevelled state of the dark-haired female protagonist and the pink ribbon (present as a garter in the 'Pamela' canvas) – may be more than coincidence. Considering the proximity in date between Highmore's 'Pamela' series (1743–44) and his association with the Foundling Hospital, demanding that the artist confront in close succession issues surrounding abuse against women and attempted rape, child abandonment and murder, it is possible that Highmore viewed the woman in *The Angel of Mercy* as representing a less fortunate Pamela, that is, one whom her 'protector' has successfully raped and then abandoned. Unlike Clarissa, here Pamela's 'other' or 'parallel' history leads her to disgrace, desolation and attempted murder. Although the renaming, during their baptism, of the infants after admission resulted in the trawling for new names from a variety of sources, including the governors themselves and popular fiction, the appearance within the General Registers of two little 'Pamela Andrews' (child 89, admitted 1741, and child 338, admitted 1747; sadly both died as infants) and one 'Clarissa Harlowe' (child 465, admitted February 1748/49; apprenticed to Joseph Isaac in 1761) poignantly brings together fact and fiction (figs. 101–03).[70]

Certainly Highmore has taken the foundling narrative of Hogarth's subscription roll design one dramatic step further. His depiction of contemporary attempted new-born child murder in progress is unique in British or even Western art. The analysis presented by Highmore in his essay 'On reputation' reveals little sympathy for the women caught up in such a scenario. Yet, as stated earlier, in the depiction of this horrific scene, some tenderness is shown towards this mother's plight: her extreme suffering is displayed through her expression and indicated by her posture. The inclusion of the angel, a figure from traditional history painting and the 'messenger' of God, is an attempt to locate Highmore's composition safely between the allegorical/biblical and contemporary worlds. In the Bible, angels bring divine communication and lead 'the chosen' away from danger to safety (as in the story of Hagar). Imminent calamity is avoided through the auspices of God via His messenger. In tandem, the 'Angel of Mercy' points, not to a miraculous spring, but towards the distinctive façade of the Foundling Hospital: in fact he does not simply indicate the presence of the Hospital, but is deliberately moving towards it.

This action is made more urgent by the angel's grip on the woman's arm and suggests that she can come willingly or by force. A single dab of paint denotes the child's protruding tongue as it slowly chokes. In

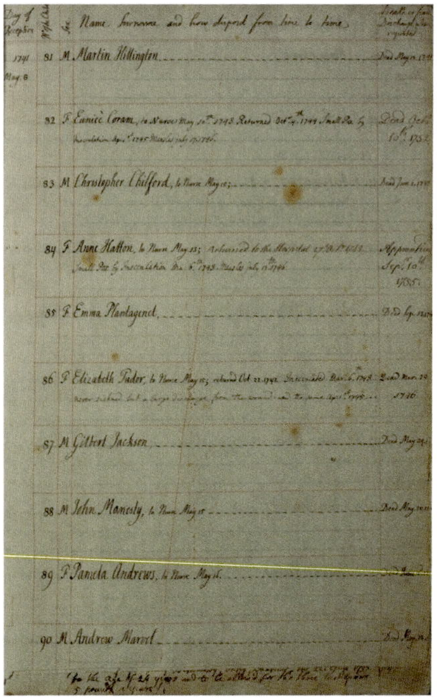
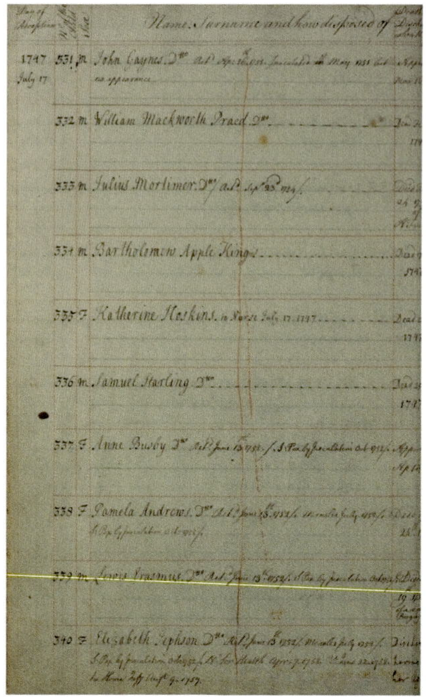
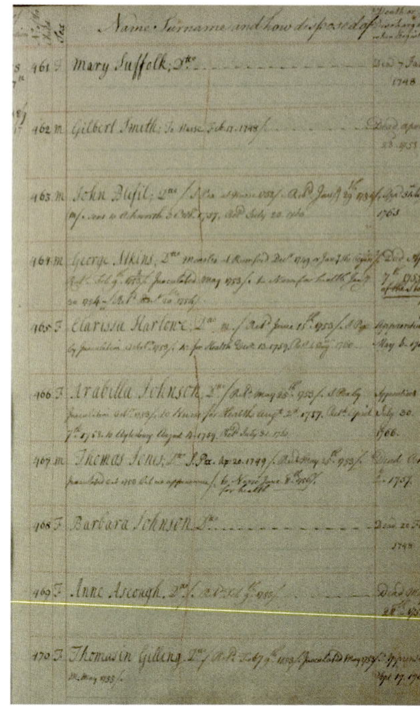

101, 102, 103 A/FH/A/09/002/001 General Register 1 (Nos 1–3595). Entries for children Nos 89 (Pamela Andrews), 338 (Pamela Andrews) and 465 (Clarissa Harlowe)

Clarissa Harlowe (no. 465) was admitted in February 1749 and named by a 'Mrs Jones' at baptism. She went to nurse on 6 October 1749 and returned to the Hospital on 15 June 1753 at the age of four years. Soon afterwards she was returned to nurse 'for health' (30 January 1754) and was then readmitted to the Hospital on 20 December 1754. She was apprenticed on 6 May 1761 to Joseph Isaac, a salesman of Middle Row, Holborn, in 'household business'. She then moved to Jane Field, a mantua maker.

such circumstances the aggressive action of the angel can be excused, indicating that, for Highmore, the absolute priority is the child. Indeed the composition and narrative of *The Angel of Mercy* quote from another popular subject from the history painting repertoire, Hercules between the personifications of Virtue and Vice, as cleverly spoofed by Hogarth in his progresses of the 'Rake' and the 'Harlot'. Here too the woman is represented at the moment of decision – to follow Virtue/Charity as represented by the angel or Vice/Cruelty as personified by the cloaked figure. One will lead to redemption of sorts, the other – in Highmore's stated opinion – damnation. These two figures, and particularly the angel, elevate a modern subject-matter into an adapted form of 'high art'. Although on one level the treatment hints at a 'modern moral subject', the references to traditional history painting are here respectful rather than satirical.[71]

However, that Highmore himself struggled to find a resolution to this complicated narrative is perhaps hinted at by the painting's unfinished state. He may have abandoned the idea as too disturbing or distasteful – a story that cannot or should not be depicted. What is striking, if we now juxtapose Highmore's treatment of the Hagar and Ishmael in the Hospital's Court Room with *The Angel of Mercy*, is the relative coyness of the former and, despite the allegorical figures, the attempted realism and honesty of the latter. This highlights the need for a sanitized depiction of the foundling story within the Governors' Court Room, despite the awareness of those involved of the multitude of real-life stories being played out in modern Britain, spanning indifference and neglect, misery and murder. Yet in *The Angel of Mercy* we can see the biblical story of Hagar and Ishmael being transformed into a very modern parable.

CONCLUSION

It is no coincidence that history painting became a visible element of Highmore's artistic output during the 1740s. The Foundling Hospital not only offered a prestigious venue for the public display of his work, but the artistic, intellectual and social stimuli to pursue it. That Highmore's gift to the Hospital dominated his professional career during the period of its creation is suggested by his known paintings for the year 1746 – three portraits and *Hagar and Ishmael* itself.[1] This dramatically reduced output implies that Highmore considered this project to be so important that he effectively took time out from his portrait practice to work on it.

A principal aim of this present study has been to reappraise Highmore's practice through the concept of variety. Although our understanding of the artist's approach to history painting is limited to three extant examples (from the fourteen ascribed to him), through analysis of these three paintings it becomes clear that Highmore viewed himself, and in the 1740s projected himself, as a painter of history as well as portraiture. The paintings analysed here, portraits, history and subject paintings, should be viewed as indicative of an artist at the peak of his career and artistic powers.

It is also clear that during the 1740s, as an artist, husband, father, citizen and 'middling sort' member of British society, Highmore was contemplating, addressing and expressing, through art and literature, some of the most controversial and pressing issues of the period; indeed, much of what concerned him then, concerns us still. The paintings discussed in this present study are at the heart of this philosophical and artistic progress. In both history painting and portraiture, Highmore is revealed as an artist employing and adapting the tools of traditional Western European painting as a means of engaging with and reflecting these contemporary contexts and issues. In the case of *The Angel of Mercy*, Highmore created one of the most original and controversial paintings in eighteenth-century British art.

Finally, Highmore emerges as an artist of greater intellect, ingenuity and importance than has hitherto been supposed, and one whose inquisitiveness, flexibility and responsiveness allowed him fully to engage with the dynamic social and cultural context within which his career developed. His example should assist in informing, or reforming, our idea of the story of British art in the early Georgian period.

NOTES

FOREWORD

1 London Metropolitan Archives A/FH/M/01/001/016.
2 Sotheby & Co., *Catalogue of Fine Paintings and Drawings of the English School*, 19 April 1961, lot 108.
3 Christie, Manson & Wood, King Street, London, *Catalogue of Important English Pictures*, Friday 7 July 1967, lot 16, illus. p. 6.
4 R. Paulson, *Hogarth, His Life, His Art and Times*, 2 vols. (New Haven and London, 1971), II, p. 44.
5 Jacqueline Riding, *Joseph Highmore 1692–1780*, 2 vols. (PhD, University of York, 2012). The supporting material was first published in the article Jacqueline Riding, '"The mere relation of the sufferings of others": Highmore, History Painting and the Foundling Hospital', *Art History*, vol. 35, no. 3 (June 2012[a]), pp. 522–53.
6 Jacqueline Riding, *Susanna Duncombe: A Quintessential Female Artist in Eighteenth-century England?* (MA dissertation, University of London, 1994). See also Jacqueline Riding, 'Susanna Duncombe', in Delia Gaze, ed., *Dictionary of Women Artists*, 2 vols. (London and Chicago, 1994), I, pp. 473–75.

'MR HIGHMORE'

1 Abraham Langford, *A Catalogue of the Genuine and Entire Collection of Pictures of Mr. Joseph Highmore* (London, 5 March 1762).
2 John Duncombe, 'Memoirs of the late Joseph Highmore, Esq', *The Gentleman's Magazine*, 50 (London, April 1780), pp. 176–79, at p. 178.
3 See British Library, Add MSS 670.38728, f. 115, Joseph Highmore's agreement to publish with John Nourse; and Royal Society Library Collections MS/597/2/33-34, letters from Joseph Highmore to John Canton, 14/29 and 19 September 1757.
4 These include *A critical examination of those two paintings on the cieling* [sic] *of the Banqueting-house at Whitehall* (London, 1754); *The Practice of Perspective, on the Principles of Dr. Brook Taylor* (London, 1763); 'On Mr Webb's Enquiry into the Beauties of Painting', *The Gentleman's Magazine*, 36 (London, August 1766[a]), pp. 353–56; 'On colouring', *The Gentleman's Magazine*, 48 (London, November 1778), pp. 526–27.
5 Langford 1762, p. 2, lot 17, and p. 4, lots 67, 68, 73 and 74.
6 Langford 1762, p. 2, lot 15.
7 Langford 1762, p. 3, lot 40, 'The Dutchess [sic] of *Hamilton*, and Lady *Coventry*'.
8 Gunning portraits are mentioned in the ode 'At the Grave of JOSEPH HIGHMORE. Esq', *St James's Chronicle* (28–30 March 1780).
9 Langford 1762, p. 3, lot 46.
10 Algernon Graves, *The Society of Artists of Great Britain etc* [1907] (Bath, 1969), p. 117, and Langford 1762, p. 4, lot 79.
11 Langford 1762, p. 2, lot 22.
12 Langford 1762, p. 2, lots 23, 24, and p. 4, lots 77 and 78.
13 Langford 1762, p. 2, lots 6 and 19.
14 Elizabeth Johnston, *Paintings by Joseph Highmore 1692–1780* (London, 1963).
15 Volume 4 now included a much larger selection of artists from the reign of George II.
16 Horace Walpole, *Anecdotes of Paintings*, 2nd edn, 4 vols. (Twickenham, 1782), IV, title page.
17 Walpole 1782, IV, pp. 121–22. The named works are the designs for the commemorative publication for the new Order of the Bath.
18 Walpole 1782, IV, p. 146.
19 J. Ireland, *Hogarth Illustrated*, 2nd edn, 3 vols. (London, 1798), I, pp. xx–xxi.
20 J.W. Scobell Armstrong, 'Joseph Highmore, painter and author', *The Connoisseur*, 86 (October 1930), pp. 209–19; C.R. Beard, 'Highmore's Scrap-book', *The Connoisseur*, vol. 93, no. 705 (1934), pp. 290–97, and 'Highmore's Drawings for Pine's Processions and Ceremonies', *The Connoisseur*, 94 (July 1934), pp. 9–15; J.W. Goodison, 'Two Portraits by Joseph Highmore', *The Burlington Magazine*, 73 (September 1938), pp. 125–27; C.H. Collins Baker, 'Joseph Highmore, Samuel Richardson, and Lady Bradshaigh', *Huntington Library Quarterly*, vol. 7, no. 3 (May 1944), pp. 316–19; F. Antal, 'Mr Oldham and his Guests by Highmore', *The Burlington Magazine*, vol. 91, no. 554 (May 1949), pp. 128–32; R. Edwards, 'Hogarth into Highmore, or a wrong redressed', *Apollo*, 90 (August 1969), pp. 148–51.
21 A.S. Lewis, *Joseph Highmore: 1692–1780. An Eighteenth Century English Portrait Painter*, 3 vols. (PhD, University of Harvard, 1975, reprinted 1976). Although the focus is portraiture, it is an important resource for the artist's life and career. It was followed by Warren Mild, *Joseph Highmore of Holborn Row* (Ardmore, 1990).
22 Elizabeth Johnston, 'Joseph Highmore's Paris Journal', *The Walpole Society*, 42 (Oxford, 1970), pp. 61–104, at p. 61.
23 Tate Archive (TGA), 866/2/1, Joseph Highmore, *Paris Journal*, 1734. It is a more comprehensive account than, for example, Sir James Thornhill's *Notebook of a visit to France*, February–April 1717 (National Art Library, MSL/1961/1455).
24 Mrs Joan Highmore Blackhall and Dr Rosemary McConnell.
25 See Jacqueline Riding, 'An Englishman in Paris: Joseph Highmore at the Académie Royale', in Hannah Williams, ed., *Journal18*, Louvre local edition (Autumn 2016[b]), www.journal18.org; 'Artistic connections between Dublin and London in the early-Georgian period: James Latham and Joseph Highmore', in Caroline Pegum and Brendan Rooney et al., eds., *Irish Fine Art in the Early Modern Period* (Dublin, 2016[a]), pp. 80–117; '*A Session of Painters*: Succession, Legacy and the prospects for British portraiture after Sir Godfrey Kneller', in Mark Hallett et al., eds., *Court, Country, City: British Art & Architecture 1660–1735* (London

and New Haven, 2016), pp. 353–79; Riding 2012[a]; 'Joseph Highmore', in *Oxford Dictionary of National Biography* (Oxford, 2004; online edition 2008, article 13247).

'AN INGENIOUS YOUNG PAINTER'

1 Duncombe 1780, p. 176.
2 *Daily Courant*, 26 November 1720.
3 I am grateful to Geoffrey Brown at Merchant Taylors' School for confirming this.
4 See H.B. Wilson, *The History of the Merchant Taylors School, from its foundation to the present*, 2 vols. (London, 1812), I, p. 11.
5 F.W.M. Draper, *Four Centuries of Merchant Taylors' School 1561–1961* (London, 1962), pp. 5–8.
6 Wilson 1812, I, p. 17.
7 Wilson 1812, II, p. 545.
8 For Spenser and Jonson see Draper 1962, pp. 31–32; for Highmore's contemporaries p. 93.
9 George Vertue Notebooks, in *The Walpole Society*, 6 vols. (Oxford, 1929–50), III, p. 29.
10 Vertue Notebooks III, p. 17.
11 Duncombe 1780, p. 176.
12 Lewis 1976, I, p. 24.
13 For Thornhill's apprenticeship with Highmore see Richard Johns, *James Thornhill and Decorative History Painting in England after 1688*, 2 vols. (PhD, University of York, 2004), I, pp. 39–40.
14 Thornhill's uncle Edward married Thomas Highmore's cousin Margaret Highmore; see Anthony Highmore Junior's footnote to 'Letter from Joseph Highmore to Sir Edward Walpole', *The Gentleman's Magazine*, 86 (London, April 1816), pp. 300–03, at p.302.
15 Vertue Notebooks III, p. 17.
16 Duncombe 1780, p. 176.
17 Duncombe 1780, p. 176.
18 Duncombe 1780, p. 177.
19 See 'Mr. Highmore' above, n. 4.
20 Andrew Wilton, *Turner in his Time* (London, 2006), p. 247. See also J.M.W. Turner, *Lecture Diagram: Perspective Method for a Cube by Joseph Highmore*, graphite and watercolour on paper, c.1823–28, 546 × 760 mm, Tate, inv. no. D16987.
21 Vertue Notebooks III, p. 17.
22 *[The] Literary Gazette, and journal of belles lettres, arts, sciences, etc* (London, 1826), p. 732.
23 Highmore 1816, p. 303.
24 Highmore 1816, p. 303.
25 Highmore 1816, p. 303.
26 Highmore included a prose translation of Isaac Hawkins Browne's Latin poem *De animi immortalitate* (first published 1754) in his *Essays, moral, religious, and miscellaneous*, 2 vols. (London, 1766), II, pp. 109–73.
27 Duncombe 1780, p. 176.
28 For a summary of the early eighteenth-century academies including membership, see Vertue Notebooks IV, pp. 168–71.
29 See Ilaria Bignamini, 'Art Institutions in London, 1689–1768. A Study of Clubs and Academies', in *The Walpole Society*, 55 (Oxford, 1988), pp. 1–148.
30 William Baxter (1650–1723), an antiquarian and schoolmaster, Dr John Gale (1680–1721), Baptist preacher and theologian, William Duncombe (1690–1769), Highmore's close friend, then a clerk in the Navy Office, and the silk merchants Moses (1679–1748) and Mathew II Raper (1665–1748).
31 Harvard University Archive, 1:15:505, quoted in P.J. Gomes, 'Thomas Hollis of London', in R.L. Petersen and C.A. Pater, eds., *The Contentious Triangle: Church, State, and University* (Missouri, 1999), p. 57.
32 *Boston News Letter*, 17 September 1751: 'To be sold by P. Pelham ... a print in Metzotintu of Thomas Hollis, late of London, merchant, a most generous Benefactor to Harvard College in New-England ... &c. done from a curious whole length Picture by Joseph Highmore in London, and placed in the College Hall in Cambridge', quoted in W.H. Whitmore, 'The Early Painters and Engravers of New England', *Proceedings of the Massachusetts Historical Society 1866–67*, 9 (1867), pp. 197–216, at p. 203.
33 Surrey History Centre BKL/1/1b/24, Little Bookham, All Saints: Parish Records, Early Registers, Marriages, 1670–1754, 28 May 1716: 'Joseph Highmore of St Swithins London & Susanna Hiller of Effingham – were married'. Susanna's father Anthony owned and leased parcels of land in the Effingham/ Bookham area of Surrey; for example, see S.H.C. K63/1/70–71, 11–12 October 1692, 'Lease and release, and bond' between 'Anthony Hiller of Effingham, yeoman' and 'Francis, Lord Howard of Effingham'.
34 For details of Anthony's life see his obituary in *The Gentleman's Magazine*, 69, pt 2 (London, October 1799), pp. 905–06.
35 Vertue Notebooks III, p. 17.
36 This is fully explored in Riding 2016, pp. 353–79.
37 Vertue Notebooks III, p. 29.
38 Duncombe 1780, p. 177.
39 Duncombe 1780, p. 177.
40 E.G. Miles, *Thomas Hudson 1701–1779* (London, 1979) no page numbers, introduction [pp. 2–4].
41 *General Advertiser*, 13 March 1749.
42 Elizabeth Carter to Susanna Highmore, 7 May 1756; transcribed in Gwen Hampshire, *Elizabeth Carter, 1717–1806. An Edition of Some Unpublished Letters* (Delaware, 2005), pp. 158–60, at p. 159.
43 For the letters from Elizabeth Carter to Susanna see Hampshire 2005, pp. 136–60, 183–85, 190–94. The 'Ariosto' drawings are Tate T04242 and T04243.
44 James Anderson, *The Constitutions of the Freemasons* (London, 1767–76), pp. 203–04, under 'Assembly and Feast at Mercers-Hall ... 27 December 1727 ... Joseph Highmore, Painter Grand Warden'.
45 G.W. Speth, ed., *Quatuor Coronatorum Antigrapha* (Margate, 1913), pp. 40–41.
46 The lodge remained in Greenwich until 1734, but by 1736 it had moved to The White Horse, Wheeler Street, Spitalfields; see under the 'United Traders' Lodge' in *Lane's Masonic Records*, www.hrionline.ac.uk/lane/.
47 Speth 1913, p. 40.
48 Highmore 1816, p. 10.
49 See National Portrait Gallery D2944. The identity of the sitter has been disputed, but he is very similar to the accepted portrait of Thornhill, NPG 4688.
50 See Speth 1913.
51 *Evening Journal*, 28 December 1727.
52 James Anderson, *The New Book of Constitutions* (London, 1738), p. 109.
53 The portrait of Sayer was still in Highmore's possession in 1762; see Langford 1762, p. 2, lot 7.
54 Duncombe 1780, p. 177.
55 For example, from 1732 to 1733 Highmore produced eight family portraits for Heneage Finch, 2nd Earl of Aylesford (1683–1757).
56 Duncombe 1780, p. 177. The Cumberland portrait was offered for sale

in 1762: see Langford 1762, p. 4, lot 66.
57 For a full exploration of both trips see Riding 2012, pp. 94–127.
58 Duncombe 1780, p. 177.
59 Henry Pemberton was author of *A View of Sir Isaac Newton's Philosophy* (London, 1728). Highmore is listed as a subscriber.
60 Langford 1762, p. 3, lots 27 and 29.
61 Highmore 1778, p. 527.
62 Jonathan Richardson (Snr) and Jonathan Richardson (Jnr), *An account of some of the statues, bas-reliefs, drawings and pictures in Italy. &c* (London, 1722), pp. 1–6.
63 Langford 1762, p. 3, lots 35 and 38, and p. 4, lots 59 and 60.
64 Rubens purchased the house and land on the Wapper in 1610.
65 Richardson and Richardson 1722, p. 351.
66 G.J. Karsch, *Designation exacte des Peintures precieuses, qui sont en grand Nombre dans la Galerie de la Residence de son Altesse Ser[me] Electorale Palatine à Dusseldorff* (Düsseldorf, 1725), nos. 162, 186, 192, 177 and 168 respectively.
67 TGA 866/2/1, 2 r and 37 v. Highmore notes that he came ashore at Dover at 11 pm on Monday 12 August.
68 See Riding 2012, I, pp. 108–14; for Daudé see pp. 111–14.
69 Riding 2012, I, pp. 108–10.
70 For Highmore at the Académie Royale see Riding 2016b.
71 TGA 866/2/1, 25r and v.
72 TGA 866/2/1, 25r.
73 TGA 866/2/1, 26r–26v.
74 Roger de Piles, *Dialogue on Colouring. Translated from the original French of M. du Pile ... by Mr Ozell* (London, 1711), pp. 36–37.
75 TGA 866/2/1, 3v–4v.
76 TGA 866/2/1, 5v.
77 TGA 866/2/1, 29v–30r.

'THE CONFIDENCE OF FRIENDSHIP ...'

1 Vertue Notebooks III, p. 29.
2 Duncombe 1780, p. 179.
3 For a thorough exploration see Kate Retford's forthcoming book, *The Conversation Piece* (2017).
4 Philippe Mercier's *The Shutz Family* of 1725 (Tate) is believed to be the first painted in England.
5 Johnston 1963, p. 28.
6 James Harris, 1st Earl of Malmesbury (1746–1820) was Harris's son.
7 John Nichols, *Literary anecdotes of the eighteenth century*, 9 vols. (London, 1812–15), III, p. 75.
8 See W.P. Baildon, *Records of the Honourable Society of Lincoln's Inn: Admissions 1420–1799*, 2 vols. (London, 1896), II, pp. 388, 393, 400 and 401.
9 Hampshire Record Office, Malmesbury Family Papers, 9M73/G605/11.
10 Sotheby's *Important Paintings by Old Masters* (New York, 15 June 1977), p. 130, lot 108.
11 Sotheby's 1977, p. 130, lot 108.
12 H.R.O. 9M73/G605/13.
13 H.R.O. 6M59/F9/1/2: John Hoadly to Richard Warner, 26 April 1744.
14 H.R.O. 9M73/G605/13.
15 Anthony Ashley-Cooper, 3rd Earl of Shaftesbury, *Characteristicks of Men, Manners, Opinions, Times*, 2 vols. (London, 1711).
16 For details of the family line see A. Collins & E. Brydges, *Collins' Peerage of England*, 9 vols. (London, 1812), V, pp. 421–22.
17 H.R.O. 9M73/G482//2: Joseph Highmore to James Harris, 5 July 1740.
18 Harris's later publications include *Three Treatises concerning Art; Music, Painting, Poetry and Happiness* (London, 1744).
19 H.R.O. 9M73/G482/3: Joseph Highmore to James Harris, 30 July 1740.
20 H.R.O. 9M73/G482/11: Joseph Highmore to James Harris, 27 March 1742.
21 H.R.O. 9M73/G482/11: Joseph Highmore to James Harris, 27 March 1742.
22 H.R.O. 9M73/G482//10: Joseph Highmore to James Harris, 23 March 1741.
23 H.R.O 9M73/G482/10: Joseph Highmore to James Harris, 23 March 1741. The double portrait mentioned is unknown.
24 See Lewis 1976, II, pp. 517–20.
25 Duncombe 1780, p. 177.
26 H.R.O. 9M73/G482/10: Joseph Highmore to James Harris, 23 March 1741.
27 See W.P. Baildon, *Records of the Honourable Society of Lincoln's Inn: The Black Books 1422–1845*, 4 vols. (London, 1897–1902), III, pp. 98 and 194.
28 Wolverhampton Art Gallery Object File: Highmore, *The Lee Family*, List of Paintings Tickencote Hall No. 44.
29 For identification of the sitters see W.A.G. Object File: Highmore, *The Lee Family*.
30 C. Gambarini, *A description of the Earl of Pembroke's Pictures* (London, 1731), p. 8.
31 S. Barnes, N. de Poorter, O. Millar and H. Vey, *Van Dyck: Complete Catalogue of Paintings* (New Haven and London, 2004), p. 572.
32 Gambarini 1731, p. 9.
33 The illustration appears to be a hybrid, i.e. 'a common Parrot', Table XVI, and 'The white crested Parrot' and "The Macao', Table XV.
34 I am grateful to the present curator, Marguerite Nugent, for confirming this.
35 For the Will of Sir Eldred Lancelot Lee of Coton dated 21 December 1732 see A. Nicholls, *The History of Alveley* (Albrighton, 1994), p. 82.
36 Re Richard Gough, 'a passage near the harbour of Chusan, in China, still bears the designation of Gough's passage': see J. Burke, *A Genealogical and Heraldic History of the Commoners of Great Britain and Ireland* (London, 1835), II, p. 394.
37 Burke 1835, II, p. 395.
38 Baildon 1896, I, II, p. 411.
39 In 1732 the painting was in the collection of Willem Six in Amsterdam; see A. Grossman, 'Holbein Studies II', *The Burlington Magazine*, 93 (April 1951), pp. 111–14, at p. 112.
40 Nicholls 1992, p. 82.
41 K. Retford, 'A Death in the Family: Posthumous Portraiture in Eighteenth-Century England', *Art History*, vol. 33, no. 1 (February 2010), pp. 74–97, at p. 82.
42 Highmore 1766, I, p. 47.
43 Letter from Lancelot Lee to the Hon. Thomas Lee, 21 May 1745; see The Lee Family Digital Archive, http://leearchive.wlu.edu/
44 Retford 2010, p. 80.
45 Retford 2010, p. 80.
46 Burke 1835, II, p. 396.
47 Engravings were available and one of several contemporary copies belonged to Watteau's patron, the comtesse de Verrue. Highmore had noted 'Verrue' in his *Paris Journal* but there is no confirmation that he visited the collection. See TGA 866/2/1, 39r.
48 The original is probably the version now in Kelvingrove Art Gallery inscribed *Magnae Matri/ Terrae omnis parenti* or 'To the Great Mother, Parent of all Earth'. It is believed to have been owned by Sir James Thornhill.
49 For the Virgin Mary see R. Verdi, *The Parrot in Art: from Dürer to Elizabeth Butterworth* (Birmingham, 2007), pp. 15–18.
50 The National Archives PROB 11/1062/357, Will of Joseph Highmore of Canterbury, Kent, proved 22 March 1780.

51 See Verdi 2007, p. 15. Marcus Valerius Martialis, or Martial (40–102/04) writes in his *Epigrammata*, LXIX 'I, a parrot, am taught by you the names of others; I have learned of myself to say, "Hail! Caesar!"': M.V. Martialis, ed. T. Fitzgerald, *Epigrammata* (London, 1721), p. 353.
52 Christopher White, *The Later Flemish Pictures in the Collection of Her Majesty the Queen* (London, 2007), pp. 23, 260.
53 Isaac Watts, *Death and Heaven or The Last Enemy Conquer'd*, 2nd edn (London, 1724), p. 62.
54 Watts 1724, pp. 34–35.
55 J. Duncombe, ed., *Letters by Several Eminent Persons Deceased including the correspondence of John Hughes*, 3 vols. (London, 1773), I, pp. 128–30.
56 Duncombe 1773, I, pp. 131–32.
57 British Library Add MSS 23,089, pp. 115–34, at p. 115.
58 See Riding 2016, pp. 372–75.
59 W. Duncombe, ed., *Poems on Several Occasions ... by John Hughes*, 2 vols. (London 1735), I, p. xxxvi.
60 A. Hadfield, *The Cambridge Companion to Spenser* (Cambridge, 2001), p. 14.
61 J. Hughes, *The Works of Mr. Edmund Spenser*, 6 vols. (London, 1715), I, pp. xxv–lvii and xxx.
62 Hughes 1715, I, p. xxxi.
63 I am grateful to Professor Andrew Hadfield for his guidance on Spenser's reception during the early eighteenth century.
64 J. Richardson, *An essay on the theory of painting* (London, 1715), pp. 190–91.
65 Hughes 1715, I, p. lxxxvi.
66 Hughes 1715, II, p. 451.
67 Hughes 1715, I, p. lxxxvi.
68 Hughes 1715, II, p. 453.
69 Hughes 1715, II, p. 454.
70 Philadelphia History Museum at the Atwater Kent.
71 J.W. Jordan, ed., *Colonial and Revolutionary Families of Pennsylvania*, 3 vols. (New York and Chicago, 1911), I, p. 6.
72 Jane Vigor, *Letters from a Lady, Who Resided Some Years in Russia, to Her Friend in England* (London, 1775), pp. 79–80.
73 See Victoria and Albert Museum T.327-2009, chair seat cover; T.323-2009, chair back cover; T.315-2009, sofa back cover.
74 Vigor 1775, pp. 88–89.
75 Vigor 1775, pp. 96–97.
76 The National Archives, State Papers Foreign, Royal Letters 102/50 Pt 1 [144–49 or 87–89], 'Translation of the Czarina's Letter to the King in favour of Mrs Rondeau', St Petersburg, 26 December 1739.
77 See K. Turner, 'Jane Vigor', *Oxford Dictionary of National Biography* (Oxford, 2004–13, online article 59244).

'HER WHOLE STORY'

1 *General Evening Post*, 16 February 1744.
2 For a recent edition see Albert J. Rivero ed., *Pamela: or, Virtue Rewarded* and *Pamela in her exalted condition* (Cambridge, 2011–12).
3 This was repeated nine further times over three weeks, and in the *Daily Advertiser* and *General Advertiser* throughout May.
4 *Daily Advertiser*, 1 May 1745.
5 *London Daily Post and General Advertiser*, 2 April 1743.
6 In 1731 Vertue noted 'near 12 hundred' subscribers for the 'Harlot' series: Vertue Notebooks III, p. 53.
7 See J.G. Turner, 'Novel Panic: Picture and Performance in the Reception of Richardson's *Pamela*', *Representations* (Autumn 1994), pp. 70–96, and Thomas Keymer and Peter Sabor, *Pamela in the Marketplace: Literary Controversy and Print Culture in Eighteenth-Century Britain and Ireland* (Cambridge, 2005).
8 *London Evening Post*, 8–11 November 1740.
9 *General Evening Post*, 16 February 1744.
10 *General Evening Post*, 16 February 1744.
11 Turner 1994, pp. 70–96, and Keymer and Sabor 2005.
12 The novel *Joseph Andrews* published in 1742 was its sequel.
13 T.C.D. Eaves, 'Graphic Illustrations of the Novels of Samuel Richardson, 1740–1810', *Huntington Library Quarterly*, vol. 14, no. 4 (August 1951), pp. 349–83, 350–51.
14 See Janet Aikins, 'Richardson's 'speaking pictures'', in Margaret Doody and Peter Sabor, eds., *Samuel Richardson Tercentenary Essays* (Cambridge, 1989), pp. 146–66, at pp. 151–52.
15 Hayman had painted Richardson and his second family c.1740–41 (Tate T12221).
16 They are the 'bundle' scene (untraced) and *Pamela fleeing from Lady Davers*: see D. Coke and A. Borg, *Vauxhall Gardens: A History* (New Haven and London, 2011), pp. 103, 368, 370–71.
17 In Keymer and Sabor 2005, p. 155, the choice is described as 'thoroughly Richardsonian'.
18 Highmore 1766, I, p. 140.
19 Samuel Richardson, *Pamela: or, Virtue Rewarded*, 6th edn, 4 vols. (London, 1742), I, p. 124.
20 Highmore describes it as 'her own little Parcel'.
21 Richardson 1742, I, p. 124.
22 Richardson 1742, I, p. v.
23 Richardson 1742, I, p. v.
24 The engraving text reads, 'Mr. B. struck with this Scene is waiting the Issue'.
25 Highmore 1766, I, p. 142.
26 *Daily Advertiser*, 3 January 1745.
27 For example *London Evening Post*, 31 January–2 February 1745. Also R. Paulson, *Hogarth*, 3 vols. (New Brunswick, 1992), II, p. 425.
28 This transcription was provided by Jocelyn Wingfield, Wingfield Family Society; see W.A.G. Object File Highmore: *The Lee Family*.
29 *The Holy Bible*, London, 1743, Proverbs 3: 27.
30 See F. Dabhoiwala, *The origins of sex: a history of the first sexual revolution* (London, 2012), pp. 141–79.
31 See M. Hallett, *The Spectacle of Difference: Graphic Satire in the Age of Hogarth* (New Haven and London, 1999), pp. 170–73.
32 For a recent discussion see M. Hallett and C. Riding, *Hogarth* (London, 2007) p. 79.
33 Richardson 1742, I, p. 174.
34 Richardson 1742, I, p. 326.
35 Richardson 1742, I, p. 341.
36 Pamela was also the subject of a series of large-scale paintings by Mercier. At least two versions are known dated c.1743–45: see J. Ingamells and R. Raines, 'A Catalogue of the Paintings, Drawings and Etchings of Philip Mercier', *The Walpole Society*, 46 (Oxford, 1978), pp. 1–70, at p. 45. But according to Alan McKillop, 'a Beautiful Print' after 'Philipp Lemercier' of 'Pamela rising from her Bed' was advertised in the *Daily Advertiser* on 21 September 1750 and therefore some years after Highmore commenced his paintings: see McKillop 1936, p. 72. This advertisement has not been traced and therefore cannot be verified.
37 E. Waterhouse, *Painting in Britain 1530–1790*, 4th edn (New Haven and London, 1994), p. 82.

38 Waterhouse 1994, p. 82.
39 See also Riding 2016b.
40 TGA 866/2/1, 26v, 'returned with Mr Hickman to Paris. dined with him Afterwards went with Mr Artau to see N Coipel and Lancret'. Also TGA 866/2/1, 30 v, 'to Car Coipel many designs one of D Quixote'.
41 See B. Allen, 'Watteau and his Imitators in Mid-Eighteenth-Century England', in F. Moureau and M.M. Grasselli, eds., *Antoine Watteau (1684–1721) le peintre, son temps et sa légende* (Paris and Geneva, 1987), pp. 259–67.
42 For example, M. Vidal, *Watteau's Painted Conversations* (New Haven and London, 1992), pp. 115–16.
43 Christie's, *Catalogue of Old Pictures and drawings* (London, 15 October 1954), p. 7, lot 35.
44 This comparison was made in Hallett and Riding 2007, p. 155.
45 Paulson 1992, II, p. 241. See also Waterhouse 1965, p. 4.
46 These engravings included *La gouvernante* (1739), *La mere laborieuse* (1740), *La Pourvoyeuse* (1742) and *Le Bénédicté* (1744).
47 *The Scullery Maid* of 1738 was sold by Geminiani in 1743; see P. Rosenberg and F. Bruyant, *Chardin* (London, 2000), pp. 230–31.
48 Among them was *The Washerwoman* of 1733 (Nationalmuseum, Stockholm): see *Mercure de France* (Paris, June 1734), p. 1405, and Rosenberg and Bruyant 2000, p. 192. See also Riding 2016b.
49 Hayman is clearly adapting a Chardin motif; see J. Carey, *Taking Time: Chardin's Boy Building a House of Cards and other paintings* (London, 2012), pp. 71–72. Truchy also engraved Hayman's *The Exercise of the See Saw* and *Leap-Frog* of 1743–44.
50 The translation is from Rosenberg and Bruyant 2000, p. 234.
51 Rosenberg and Bruyant 2000, pp. 32 and 234.
52 See Rosenberg and Bruyant 2000 and Carey 2012.
53 '*Le succés des romans anglais, rapidement traduits en français ou présentés en version bilingue dès leur parution, a permis de faire conaître en France les peintres anglais qui les ont illustrés. Il en fut ainsi pour le peintre Joseph Highmore, l'illustrateur de Pamela de Richardson en 1741*': M. Polge, 'William Hogarth, sa reception par les Français au XVIIIe siécle', *The British Art Journal*, vol. 7, no. 2 (2006), pp. 12–23, at p. 16. For a discussion of Pamela's success in France see L. Festa, 'Sentimental Bonds and Revolutionary Characters: Richardson's *Pamela* in England and France' in M. Cohen and C. Dever, eds., *The Literary Channel: The Inter-National Invention of the Novel* (Princeton and Oxford, 2002) pp. 73–105.
54 This translation was kindly provided by Juliet Carey.
55 T.C.D. Eaves, 'Graphic Illustrations of the Novels of Samuel Richardson, 1740–1810', *Huntington Library Quarterly*, vol. 14, no. 4 (August 1951), p. 357.
56 F. Basan, *Dictionaire de graveurs anciens et moderns avec une notice des principales estampes*, 2 vols. (Paris, 1767), II, p. 513.
57 Highmore 1766, I, pp. 168–95, at p. 174.
58 Highmore 1766, I, pp. 94–195.
59 Highmore 1766, I, p. 175; *The Holy Bible* 1743, Proverbs 30: 8.
60 For example T. Eagleton, *The Rape of Clarissa: Writing, Sexuality and Class Struggle in Samuel Richardson* (Minneapolis, 1982).
61 'O Skilful Highmore! Can thy noble art/ Express the beauties of a worthy heart?/ Canst thou such dazzling colours blend,/ As may to future ages shew/ The whole of thy illustrious friend,/ And bid each virtue on thy canvas glow?': Thomas Mulso, *Ode to Mr. Highmore, on Mr. Richardson's sitting to him for his Picture*, in A.L. Barbauld, *The Correspondence of Samuel Richardson*, 6 vols. (London 1804), V, pp. 286–88.
62 L. Shepherd, *Clarissa's Painter: Portraiture, Illustration, and Representation in the Novels of Samuel Richardson* (Oxford, 2009), p. 105.
63 Richardson was a regular correspondent with Susanna; see Barbauld 1804, II, pp. 203–57, 280–93, 308–11.
64 Barbauld 1804, IV, p. 255.
65 Samuel Richardson, *Clarissa: Or the history of a young lady*, 7 vols. (London, 1748), III, p. 259. This painting is untraced. In 1887 John Everett Millais painted 'Clarissa' in the style of Thomas Gainsborough's *The Hon. Mrs Graham* (1775, National Galleries of Scotland), wearing a peach silk 'Van Dyck' dress (private collection).
66 Richardson 1748, VII, p. 303.
67 See Tate Collections T04195, T04196 and T04194.
68 Langford 1762, p. 2.
69 Richardson 1748, III, pp. 259–60.
70 Barbauld 1804, IV, p. 249, 6–11 January 1749 [1748/49].
71 Barbauld 1804, IV, pp. 255–56, October 1749?; Peter Sabor, ed., *Correspondence of Samuel Richardson* (Cambridge, 2016) V, pp. 66–67.
72 Barbauld 1804, IV, pp. 359–60, 15 February 1749/50; Sabor 2016, V, p. 117.
73 Barbauld 1804, IV, p. 347, 17 February 1749/50.
74 Barbauld 1804, IV, p. 360; Sabor 2016, V, p. 117. John and his wife Mary are named in Highmore's will regarding a legacy of £10.
75 Barbauld 1804, IV, p. 350; Sabor 2016, V, p. 112.
76 Barbauld 1804, VI, pp. 23–24, letter dated 3 June 1750.
77 *The Gentleman's Magazine*, 36 (London, February 1766), p. 83.
78 Grimes is now thought to be Thomas Lumley, later 3rd Earl of Scarborough; see Sabor 2016, V, p. 46.
79 T.C. Muilman, *An Apology for the conduct of Mrs T. C. Phillips, more particularly that part of it which relates to her marriage with an eminent Dutch Merchant (H. Muilman), etc*, 3 vols. (London, 1748–49), I, pp. 44–45.
80 *The Gentleman's Magazine*, 18 (London, November 1748), p. 528, and *The Gentleman's Magazine*, 19 (London, February 1749), p. 96.
81 Barbauld 1804, IV, p. 237.
82 *Old England*, Saturday 16 July 1748.
83 Langford 1762, p. 3, 'Half Lengths', lot 48, 'The original Picture of *Constantia Phillips*; from which the mezzotinto Print was taken'.
84 National Art Library FM XV, 2, f. 86, letter from Joseph Highmore to Samuel Richardson [Autumn 1747], quoted in T. Keymer, *Richardson's Clarissa and the Eighteenth-Century Reader* (Cambridge 1992), pp. 165–66.
85 The 'Clementina' full-length portrait was exhibited at the Free Society of Artists' exhibition in 1761; see Graves [1907] 1969, p. 117.
86 Langford 1762, p. 4, lots 77 and 78.
87 [T. Brecknock], 'Captain Cockade', *The Important triflers. A satire: set forth in a journal of pastime a-la-mode* (London, 1748), p. 12.

'THE SUFFERINGS OF OTHERS'

1 This chapter is an adapted and expanded version of Riding 2012, I, pp. 221–54, and Riding 2012a.
2 A. Félibien and A. Testelin, trans., *Seven conferences held in the King of France's cabinet of paintings* (London, 1740), pp. xxvii-xxviii.
3 In addition to Langford 1762 and Duncombe 1780, see J. Greenwood, *A Catalogue of a collection of pictures ...* (London, 1785), p. 7, 'Charles the 1st at Titchfield, taken by Hammond', and G.H. Robins, *Sir Walter Stirling Sale Catalogue* (London, 12–18 July 1826), p. 56, lot 92, 'A fine painting of Christ with the Disciples at Emmaus' and p. 65, lot 236, 'Virgin and Child with St John, after Raphael'. The last two paintings were from a group of 22 works by Highmore in the Stirling sale. Whitley observed that 'Sir Walter must have had a particular admiration for the works of Highmore ... in view of his increasing importance in the sale-room, I give the titles of them all': W.T. Whitley, *Art in England 1821–1837* (Cambridge, 1930), pp. 110–11.
4 *The Holy Bible* 1743., Gospel of St Luke 10: 33-34.
5 *The Holy Bible* 1743, Gospel of St Luke 10: 36.
6 T. Stackhouse, *A New History of the Holy Bible*, 2nd edn, 2 vols. (London, 1742–44), II, p. 1363, n. 5.
7 Stackhouse 1742–44, II, p. 1364.
8 I. Watts, *A Preservative from the Sins and Follies of Childhood and Youth*, 5th edn (London, 1743), p. 31.
9 J. Highmore, *Observations on a Pamphlet entitled "Christianity not founded on Argument"* (London, 1765) title page.
10 Highmore 1765, p. 1.
11 Highmore 1765, p. 1.
12 Highmore 1765, p. 11.
13 Duncombe 1780, p. 178. For Sheppard see W.M. Roberts, *Lost Country Houses of Suffolk* (Woodbridge, 2010), p. 47.
14 Garrold, Turner & Son, *A Catalogue of the Sale at Campsey Ashe High House* (Ipswich, 1-4 October 1883), p. 25; see also Tate Gallery Records, A23287 60a/04/5C, 'Joseph Highmore', and Einberg and Egerton 1988, pp. 60–62.
15 Little is known of the seventeenth-century house. There is no mention of a chapel in the brief survey in Roberts 2010, pp. 47–49.
16 The victim's 'classical' physique is based on the Belvedere Torso; see Highmore's drawings Tate T04233 and T04234.
17 Einberg and Egerton 1988, p. 60.
18 Vertue Notebooks III, p. 131.
19 For example, 'One suspects it was Hogarth once more who laid down the iconographic programme for the pictorial decoration of the Court Room': Benedict Nicholson, *The Treasures of the Foundling Hospital* (Oxford, 1972), p. 25.
20 The hospitals depicted are: Charterhouse (Thomas Gainsborough), St George's and the Foundling (Richard Wilson), Chelsea and Bethlem (Edward Haytley), St Thomas's, Christ's and Greenwich (Samuel Wale).
21 See Brian Allen, 'The East India Company Settlement pictures by George Lambert and Samuel Scott', in P. Rohatgi and P. Pheroza Godrej, eds., *Under the Indian Sun: British Landscape Artists* (Bombay, 1995), pp. 1–16; Alan Borg, 'Theodore Jacobsen and the building of the Foundling Hospital', *The Georgian Society Journal*, 13 (2003), pp. 12–53. Borg argues the Court Room scheme was Jacobsen's idea.
22 Daniel Defoe, *The Generous Projector, or a Friendly Proposal to prevent Murder and other enormous Abuses, by erecting an Hospital for Foundlings and Bastard-Children etc, London* (London, 1731), p. iv.
23 J.-A. Rouquet, *The present state of the arts in England* (London, 1755), pp. 21-33, at p. 22.
24 Rouquet 1755, pp. 25–26.
25 [Anon.], *An Account of the Hospital for the Maintenance & Education of exposed & deserted Young Children* (London, 1749), p. xiv.
26 After sizable legacies to friends and relations, 'All the rest and residue of his estate, consisting of freehold copyhold and leasehold messuages land tenements ready money plate jewels rings monies due to him from the Government monies in public stocks and monies due from any other sources, to the said Governors and Guardians of the Hospital for exposed and deserted young children and to their successors and assigns forever': The National Archives PROB 11/748, signed 4 January 1746, proved London 17 July 1746.
27 *The Gentleman's Magazine* 16 (London, July 1746), p. 383; *The London Magazine: Or, Gentleman's Monthly Intelligencer*, 15 (London, July 1746), p. 370; *Westminster Journal or New Weekly Miscellany*, 12 July 1746, p. 4.
28 David H. Solkin, *Painting for Money* (New Haven and London, 1992), pp. 157–74.
29 Highmore 1766, II, pp. 2–3.
30 'Narrative; tale; account ... recital of facts', in Samuel Johnson, *A dictionary of the English language*, 2 vols. (London, 1755), p. 2.
31 George Turnbull, *A Treatise on Ancient Painting* (London, 1740), p. 141.
32 General Court Minutes, 31 December 1746, quoted in Nicholson 1972, p. 20.
33 *Universal Spectator and Weekly Journal*, 21 March 1730, p. 3, and *Daily Advertiser*, 15 June 1731, p. 1.
34 *The Holy Bible* 1743, Book of Genesis 21: 16.
35 *The Holy Bible* 1743, Book of Genesis 21: 17.
36 For example Adriaen van der Werff, *Sarah presenting Hagar to Abraham*, 1696 (Hermitage Museum, St Petersburg).
37 Examples include Pier Francesco Mola, *The Angel appearing to Hagar and Ishmael in the Desert* 1657 (Musée du Louvre, Paris), which by 1727 was in the collection of Philippe, duc d'Orléans at the Palais-Royal, a collection Highmore visited several times in 1734, and Charles Le Brun, *Hagar and Ishmael in the Desert* (now untraced), engraved by Bernard Picart in 1707.
38 D.S. Allin, *The Early Years of the Foundling Hospital 1739/41–1773* (London, 2010), p. 387.
39 A. Levene, *Childcare, health and mortality at the London Foundling Hospital 1741–1800* (Manchester, 2007), p. 18.
40 J. Styles, *Threads of Feeling: The London Foundling Hospital's Textile Tokens, 1740–1770* (London, 2010), p. 17.
41 The petition is transcribed in R.H. Nichols and F.A. Wray, *The History of the Foundling Hospital* (London, 1935), p. 16.
42 A. Nolan, *Philanthropy and Visual Culture in Mid-Eighteenth-Century Britain: The Public Image of the London Foundling Hospital, 1739–1760* (PhD, University of East Anglia, 2002) p. 261.
43 Nolan 2002, pp. 262–63.
44 *The Holy Bible* 1743, Gospel of St Mark 10: 14.
45 Nichols and Wray 1935, pp. 15–16.
46 Matthew Henry, *An exposition of all the books of the Old and New Testamentt*, 6 vols. (London 1721–25), I, p. 74.
47 The most recent example is David H. Solkin, *Art in Britain 1660–1815* (New Haven and London, 2015), p. 103.

48 Regarding the Foundling Hospital, Solkin omits those by Highmore and Wills, while Hayman's is only named; see Solkin 2015, p. 103.

49 John Brownlow, *Memoranda: or, Chronicles of the Foundling Hospital* (London, 1847), p. 15.

50 [Anon.] 1749, p. xiv, and Rouquet 1755, p. 26.

51 [Anon.] 1749, pp. ix-x.

52 Toni Bowers, *The Politics of Motherhood: British writing and culture, 1680–1760* (Cambridge, 1996), p. 13; Hallett and Riding 2007, p. 206.

53 [Anon.] 1749, pp. ix–x.

54 Rouquet 1755, p. 26.

55 See M. Jackson, *New-Born Child Murder: Women, illegitimacy and the courts in eighteenth-century England* (Manchester, 1996).

56 'Married women and men were apparently infrequently suspected and certainly rarely indicted'; see Jackson 1996, p. 3.

57 *The Proceedings of the Old Bailey Online* (2015): www.oldbaileyonline.org reference number t17300828-28.

58 *Proceedings of the Old Bailey Online* reference number t17340630-17.

59 According to the records across England in the eighteenth century, most accused were acquitted; see Jackson 1996, p. 3.

60 *Proceedings of the Old Bailey Online* reference number t17350116-11.

61 A. Highmore, *Pietas Londinensis* (London, 1814), p. 717.

62 Styles 2010, pp. 43–51.

63 See G. Clark, 'Infant Clothing in the Eighteenth Century: A New Insight', *Costume*, vol. 28, no. 1 (1994), pp. 47–59. I am very grateful to Janette Bright for collating this data.

64 C. Ripa, *Iconologia* (Rome, 1603), p. 99.

65 Reported on 5 October 1745; see Jacqueline Riding, *Jacobites: A New History of the '45 Rebellion* (London, 2016), pp. 213–14.

66 Highmore 1766, II, p. 8.

67 General Committee Minutes A/FH/K/02/001 13 December 1739.

68 Henry Fielding, *The History of Tom Jones: A Foundling*, 6 vols. (London, 1749), I, pp. 13–14.

69 Only the west wing existed in October 1745 but the designs were agreed in 1742 and engravings existed prior to its completion.

70 My thanks again to Janette Bright for collating this information.

71 See Hallett & Riding 2007, pp. 73–94, 141–58; Elizabeth Einberg, *William Hogarth* (New Haven and London, 2016) pp. 133–41.

CONCLUSION

1 *Duchess of Chandos* (Walker Art Gallery), *Thomas Ripley* (NPG), *Mary Prenn and Dorothy Blackwell* (Musée Jacquemart-André).

FURTHER READING

Brian Allen, *Francis Hayman* (New Haven, 1987)

Louise Curran, *Samuel Richardson and the Art of Letter-Writing* (Cambridge, 2016)

Elizabeth Einberg, *Manners & Morals: Hogarth and British Painting 1700-1760* (London, 1987)

Elizabeth Einberg and Judy Egerton, *The Age of Hogarth* (London, 1988)

Mark Hallett & Christine Riding, *Hogarth* (London, 2006)

Caro Howell, *The Foundling Museum: An Introduction*, (London, 2014)

Mark Jackson, *New-Born Child Murder: Women, illegitimacy and the courts in eighteenth-century England* (Manchester, 1996)

Ruth McClure, *Coram's Children: London Foundling Hospital in the Eighteenth Century* (New Haven, 1981)

Benedict Nicolson, *The Treasures of the Foundling Hospital* (Oxford, 1972)

Roy Porter, *Enlightenment: Britain and the Creation of the Modern World* (London, 2001)

Kate Retford, *The Art of Domestic Life: Family Portraiture in Eighteenth-Century England* (New Haven, 2006)

John Styles, *Threads of Feeling: The London Foundling Hospital's Textile Tokens 1740-1779* (London, 2010)

William Vaughan, *British Painting: The Golden Age* (London, 1999)

Gillian Wagner, *Thomas Coram, Gent., 1668-1751* (Martlesham, 2004)

INDEX OF NAMES

Page numbers are followed by figure numbers in bold

PHOTOGRAPHIC CREDITS

Figs. 1, 2, 3, 5, 10, 11, 14, 17, 18, 54, 66, 82, 83 © Tate, London 2016; figs. 4, 74, 78, 79, 80, 84 © National Portrait Gallery, London; fig. 6 Private Collection. Bridgeman Images; figs. 7, 8, 9, 49, 59, 70 © National Gallery of Victoria, Melbourne; figs. 12, 13, 16, 24, 76, 87, 88, 94, 97, 99 Yale Center for British Art, Paul Mellon Collection; fig. 15 © Art Gallery of South Australia, Adelaide; fig. 19 © National Trust, Waddesdon Manor; fig. 20 © National Trust Images; figs. 21, 55, 56, 57, 58, 60, 62 Courtesy of the Garrick Club, London; fig. 22 By kind permission of the Earl of Malmesbury; fig. 23 Photo © Christie's Images / Bridgeman Images; fig. 25 © Wolverhampton Art Gallery; fig. 26 Collection of the Earl of Pembroke, Wilton House, Wilts. / Bridgeman Images; fig. 27 © The National Gallery, London; figs. 28, 100 © Metropolitan Museum of Art, New York; fig. 29 © Museo Nacional del Prado; fig. 30 © CSG CIC Glasgow Museums and Libraries Collections; figs. 31, 52, 63, 72 © The Fitzwilliam Museum, Cambridge; fig. 32 Royal Collection Trust / © HM Queen Elizabeth II 2017; fig. 33 © Victoria and Albert Museum, London; fig. 34 © The Trustees of the British Museum; figs. 35–45, 47, 50, 53, 61, 68 Yale Center for British Art, Yale Art Gallery Collection, Gift of the Library Associates; figs. 46, 48, 51 The William Ready Division of Archives and Research Collections, McMaster University Library; fig. 64 © Historic England Archive; fig. 66 Scottish National Gallery. Bequest of Lady Murray of Henderland 1861. Photographer Antonia Reeve; fig. 67 Photo: The National Gallery Library, London; fig. 68 © Photo SCALA, Florence; fig. 71 © The Hunterian, University of Glasgow 2017; fig. 73Worshipful Company of Stationers & Newspapermakers, UK. Bridgeman Images; fig. 75 © The Morgan Library and Museum, New York; fig. 77 Detroit Institute of Arts, USA. Gift of Mr and Mrs Frederick S. Ford in memory of John B. Ford. Bridgeman Images; fig. 81 Courtesy of St Bartholomew's Hospital Archives; figs. 85, 86, 89–92, 95, 96, 98, 101, 101, 102 © Coram, in the care of the Foundling Museum; fig. 93 © Country Life